PENGUIN HEALTH

LIVING WITH STRESS

Cary L. Cooper is currently Professor of Organizational Psychology at the University of Manchester Institute of Science and Technology. He is an American who has lived in Britain for twenty years and has become particularly well known over here through his Channel 4 series *How to Survive the 9 to 5*, a programme about stress that gained record viewing figures. Professor Cooper is the author of numerous books, mainly on the subject of stress at work. He has written over 200 articles for academic journals, and is a frequent contributor to newspapers including the *Guardian*, the *Daily Telegraph*, *The Times* and the *International Herald Tribune* on topics of managerial and organizational behaviour. He is Editor of the international *Journal of Organizational Behavior* and has been an adviser to two United Nations agencies: the World Health Organization and the International Labour Office, in the area of occupational stress.

Rachel Davies Cooper obtained her Ph.D. from the Institute of Advanced Studies at Manchester Polytechnic. She has carried out a number of research projects and has published in the areas of graphic design, the printing industry, and design management. In addition, she has collaborated on numerous studies with her husband, Professor Cary Cooper, in the occupational stress and health fields, and has published a number of scholarly articles in these areas. She is currently Research Fellow at Salford College of Salford University.

Lynn Hamilton Eaker obtained her undergraduate degree in journalism from the University of Oklahoma and her MBA from Southern Methodist University. She was Assistant City Editor of the *Daily Oklahoma*, and was Corporate Planner at the Republic of Texas Corporation.

CARY L. COOPER,
RACHEL D. COOPER,
LYNN H. EAKER

LIVING WITH STRESS

PENGUIN BOOKS

PENGUIN BOOKS

Published by the Penguin Group
Penguin Books Ltd, 27 Wrights Lane, London W8 5TZ, England
Penguin Books USA Inc., 375 Hudson Street, New York, New York 10014, USA
Penguin Books Australia Ltd, Ringwood, Victoria, Australia
Penguin Books Canada Ltd, 10 Alcorn Avenue, Toronto, Ontario, Canada M4V 3B2
Penguin Books (NZ) Ltd, 182–190 Wairau Road, Auckland 10, New Zealand

Penguin Books Ltd, Registered Offices: Harmondsworth, Middlesex, England

First published 1988
10 9 8 7

Printed in England by Clays Ltd, St Ives plc
Filmset in Monophoto Sabon

CONTENTS

ACKNOWLEDGEMENTS

We would like to thank all the researchers working in the stress field who have made this book possible. We would particularly like to point out the major contributions to our understanding of stress: Jim and Jonathan Quick, Martin Shaffer, Jack Ivancevich, Karl Albrecht, Andrew Melhuish, Leon Warshaw, Alan McLean, and many others.

We would also like to thank our secretary, Betty Dempsey, for her patience and help with the preparation of this book.

PREFACE

We have attempted in this volume to highlight the various aspects of the nature, dynamics and processes of stress, or what we term as the 'stress equation'. The stress equation is comprised of the source of stress at work and in life generally, together with an individual's personality characteristics (such as vulnerability), which then results in stress symptoms and, ultimately, more serious outcomes.

Life Stress + Work Stress + Individual Vulnerability = Stress Symptoms/Outcomes

In the first five chapters in this book, you should be able to identify your own components of the stress equation. Chapters 6 and 7 provide the reader with ideas, methods and techniques of coping with the stress agents identified in the earlier chapters.

- Chapter 1 helps you identify your own symptoms of stress.
- Chapter 2 highlights the various individual and organizational stress outcomes and costs.
- Chapter 3 enables you to assess your own personal vulnerability to stress.
- Chapter 4 helps you to identify your stress agents at work.
- Chapter 5 indicates sources of stress at home and in your personal life.
- Chapter 6 provides strategies and methods of dealing with work stress.
- Chapter 7 highlights coping strategies of handling stressful personal and home/life issues.

Chapter One

WHAT IS STRESS?

'A slow sort of country!' said the Queen. 'Now here, you see, it takes all the running you can do, to keep in one place. If you want to get somewhere else, you must run at least twice as fast as that!'

Lewis Carroll, *Through the Looking Glass*

Stress – this six-letter word has found as firm a place in our modern vocabularies as 'fast foods' and 'software packages'. We toss the term about casually to describe a wide range of ills resulting from our hectic pace: 'I really feel stressed,' someone says to describe a vague yet often acute sense of ailing. 'She's under a lot of stress,' we say when trying to understand a colleague's irritability or forgetfulness. 'It's a high-stress job,' someone says, awarding an odd sort of prestige to certain occupations. But to those whose ability to cope with day-to-day matters is at a crisis point, the concept of stress is no longer a casual one; for them, stress can be translated into a four-letter word: pain.

Despite the current popularity of the idea of stress, researchers and academics have long attempted to understand the causes of stress and its effects upon people. Increasingly they are trying to answer the following questions: what is stress? Why and when is stress harmful? Why do some people seem to cope so much better than others with the pressures of their lives? And finally, can people be taught the skills necessary to cope with stress?

A DEFINITION OF STRESS

Stress is a word derived from the Latin word *stringere*, meaning to draw tight, and was used in the seventeenth century to describe hardships, or affliction. During the late eighteenth century, stress denoted 'force, pressure, strain or strong effort', referring primarily to an individual, or to the individual's organs or mental powers.[1]

Early definitions of strain and load used in physics and engineering eventually came to influence one concept of how stress affects individuals. Under this concept, external forces (load) are seen as exerting pressure upon an individual, producing strain. Proponents of this view indicate we can measure the stress to which an individual is subjected in the same way we can measure physical strain upon a machine.

While this first concept looked at stress as an outside stimulus, a second concept defines stress as a person's response to a disturbance. As early as 1910, Sir William Osler explored the idea of stress and strain causing 'disease', when he saw a relationship between chest pains (angina pectoris) and a hectic pace of life. The idea that environmental forces could actually cause disease rather than just short-term ill effects, and that people have a natural tendency to resist such forces, was seen in the work of Walter B. Cannon in the 1930s. Cannon studied the effects of stress upon animals and people, and in particular studied the 'fight or flight' reaction. Through this reaction, people, as well as animals, will choose whether to stay and fight or try to escape when confronting extreme danger. Cannon observed that when his subjects experienced situations of cold, lack of oxygen, and excitement, he could detect physiological changes such as emergency adrenalin secretions. Cannon described these individuals as being 'under stress'.

One of the first scientific attempts to explain the process of stress-related illness was made by physician and scholar Hans Selye,[2] who in 1946 described three stages an individual encounters in stressful situations:

1 *Alarm Reaction*, in which an initial phase of lowered resistance is followed by countershock, during which the individual's defence mechanisms become active;
2 *Resistance*, the stage of maximum adaptation and, hopefully, successful return to equilibrium for the individual. If, however, the stress agent continues or the defence mechanism does not work, he will move on to a third stage;
3 *Exhaustion*, when adaptive mechanisms collapse.

Critics of Selye's work say it ignores both the psychological impact of stress upon an individual, and the individual's ability to recognize stress and act in various ways to change his or her situation.

Newer and more complete theories of stress emphasize the interaction between a person and his or her environment. Stress is described by one researcher as a 'response to internal or external processes' which reach levels that strain physical and psychological capacities 'to, or beyond, their limit'.[3]

In the 1970s, psychologist Richard S. Lazarus suggested that an individual's stress reaction 'depends on how the person interprets or appraises (consciously or unconsciously) the significance of a harmful, threatening or challenging event'. Lazarus's work disagrees with those who see stress simply as environmental pressure. Instead, the intensity of the stress experience is determined significantly by how well a person feels he can cope with an identified threat. If a person is unsure of his coping abilities, he is likely to feel helpless and overwhelmed.[4]

Similarly, Tom Cox in the late 1970s rejected the idea of looking at stress as simply either environmental pressures or as physiological responses. He and his fellow researchers suggest that stress can best be understood as 'part of a complex and dynamic system of transaction between the person and his environment'. Cox criticized the mechanical model of stress: 'Men and their organizations are not machines . . . Stress has to be perceived or recognized by man. A machine, however, does not have to recognize the load or stress placed upon it.'[5]

By looking at stress as resulting from a misfit between an individual and his particular environment, as will be done throughout this book, we can begin to understand why one person seems to flourish in a certain setting, while another suffers. Researchers Tom Cummings and Cary Cooper have designed a way of understanding the stress process, which can be explained thus:

- Individuals, for the most part, try to keep their thoughts, emotions and relationships with the world in a 'steady state'.
- Each factor of a person's emotional and physical state has a 'range of stability', in which that person feels comfortable. On the other hand, when forces disrupt one of these factors beyond

the range of stability, the individual must act or cope to restore a feeling of comfort.

- An individual's behaviour aimed at maintaining a steady state makes up his 'adjustment process', or coping strategies.

Included in the above description of the stress process are the ideas described below.

A stress is any force that puts a psychological or physical factor beyond its range of stability, producing a strain within the individual. Knowledge that a stress is likely to occur constitutes a threat to the individual. A threat can cause a strain because of what it signifies to the person.[6] This description can be summarized in Figure 1.

As can be seen throughout this chapter, the idea of stress and its effects upon people has evolved from different research perspectives. Figure 2 summarizes these different approaches into a general overview of the concept of stress.

Stress is clearly part of the human condition. Because of its universal presence, stress is not looked at in terms of its presence or absence in this book, but rather according to its degree and the effect it has upon individuals. Many of us seem to cope well with the pressures of work and family life encountered daily. But when and why is stress harmful to us? Consider what happens to the human body when it is subjected to a strain or pressure of some kind.

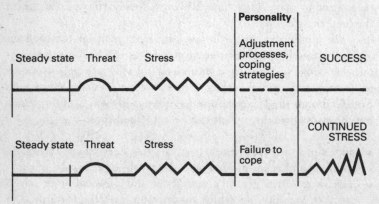

Figure 1. The Cooper–Cummings Framework

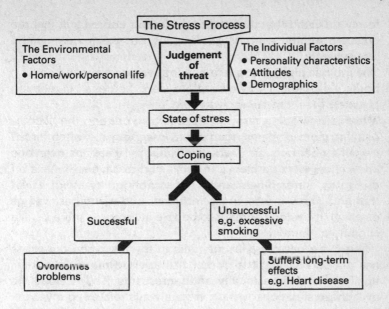

Figure 2. The Stress Process

SYMPTOMS OF STRESS

'I get frequent upset stomachs which I know are directly related to my job. Indeed, as soon as I know I have to see my boss about something, I find it hard to cope and feel my stomach grip.'

'I get very, very tired. I go to bed but sometimes I wake up in the middle of the night and think of all the things that should have been done and which I haven't done.'

'I seem to eat like a pig when I am under stress at work. When there are deadlines and pressures on me from my boss, I put on pounds!'

'When I first became a supervisor, I smoked more and sometimes I would come home and bawl my eyes out. I used to say to my husband that it's too much, I can't cope. I still feel the pressure and the symptoms still occur, but less frequently and less severely.'

'My job has given me severe headaches and frequently crying bouts. I also find it very difficult to sleep before a big meeting or when I feel I'm being evaluated.'

'When I was going through trouble at work and the accompanying stomach pains, even when I was very ill, I often forced myself to come in so I wouldn't look as weak, as everyone knew there were problems. In fact I had to have six weeks off due to my stress illness and I felt terribly guilty about it. Although I knew it was stress-induced, and mental as well as physical, I wouldn't admit it to people at work . . . there's still a stigma you know!'

'There have been regular intervals in my life when the stress has got so bad that the doctor has advised me to take tranquillizers, and occasionally antidepressants. They helped me over these situations, which were always related to my work problems.'

As Andrew Melhuish, a physician specializing in stress, has suggested, man is the product of many thousands of years of evolution and for him to survive required a quick physical response to dangers. His body 'developed the ability to rev-up' for a short time.' Walter Cannon described this mobilization of forces as the 'fight or flight' reaction mentioned earlier. Primitive man expended this burst of energy and strength in physical activity, such as a life and death struggle or a quick dash to safety.

Modern man has retained his hormonal and chemical defence mechanisms through the centuries. But for the most part, our lifestyle today does not allow physical reaction to the stress agents we face. Attacking the boss, slugging an insolent clerk or smashing an empty automatic cash dispenser are not solutions allowed by today's society. (Although such physical responses would create even more problems for most people in real life, it is interesting to note the vicarious appeal of violent physical acts in television and movies for a large part of our modern population.) Today, even the non-aggressive 'flight' reaction hardly would be judged appropriate in most situations. The executive who flees from a tense meeting, and the assembly worker who dashes out in the middle of a shift, will likely suffer the consequences of their actions. Our long-evolved defence mechanisms prepare us for dramatic and rapid action, but find little outlet. The body's strong chemical and hormonal responses are then like frustrated politicians: All dressed up with nowhere to go.

It is this waste of our natural response to stress which may actually harm us. Although scientists do not fully understand this process, it is believed that our thought patterns regarding ourselves and the situations we are in trigger events within the two branches of our central nervous system, the 'sympathetic' and the 'parasympathetic'. As researcher Karl Albrecht describes it, in a situation of challenge, tension or pressure, the sympathetic nervous system 'comes into play and activates a virtual orchestra of hormone secretions'. It is through this activation that the hypothalamus, when recognizing a danger, triggers the pituitary gland. The pituitary releases hormones, causing the adrenal glands to intensify the output of adrenalin into the bloodstream. This adrenalin, along with corticosteroid hormones released through the same process enhances one's level of arousal. All these stress chemicals stimulate the cognitive, neurological, cardiovascular, and muscular systems.[8]

These physiological changes are designed to improve the individual's performance: blood supply to the brain is increased, initially improving judgement and decision-making; the heart speeds up, increasing blood supply to the muscles, and breathing rate and function improve; glucose and fats are released into the bloodstream to provide additional energy.[9] As part of these physical changes, blood pressure rises, and blood is drained from the stomach and intestines, as well as the skin, resulting in the cold hands and feet often associated with a nervous disposition.

While these changes are the result of the role of the sympathetic branch, the parasympathetic branch can induce a state of relaxation and tranquillity. As Albrecht notes, 'people who have spent much of their time in an over-anxious or tense state have difficulty in bringing into action the parasympathetic branch' and

Table 1.
Effects of Pressure on Bodily Functions

	Normal – Relaxed	Under Pressure
Brain	Blood supply normal	Blood supply increases
Mood	Happy	Serious
Saliva	Normal	Reduced
Muscles	Blood supply normal	Blood supply increases
Heart	Normal heart rate and blood pressure	Output rate and blood pressure increases
Lungs	Normal respiration	Respiration rate increases
Stomach	Normal blood supply and acid secretion	Blood supply decreases acid secretion increases
Bowels	Normal blood supply and bowel activity	Blood supply decreases motility increases
Bladder	Normal function	Frequent micturition
Sexual organs	(M) Normal sex (F) Normal periods, etc	(M) Impotence (blood supply decreases) (F) Irregular periods
Skin	Healthy	Dry skin, blood supply decreases
Biochemistry	Normal, oxygen consumed, glucose and fats liberated	Oxygen consumption increases, glucose and fat consumption increases

Source: A. Melhuish; *Executive Health* (London: Business Books), 1978

Acute Pressure	Chronic Pressure (Stress)
Thinks more clearly	Headaches and migraines, tremor and nervous tics
Increased concentration	Anxious and loses sense of humour
Reduced	Dry mouth, lump in throat
Improved performance	Muscular tension and pain
Improved performance	Hypertension and chest pain
Improved performance	Coughs and asthma
Reduced blood supply reduces digestion	Heartburn and indigestion giving ulcers
Reduced blood supply reduces digestion	Abdominal pain and diarrhoea
Increased nervous stimulation gives frequency	Frequency and prostatic symptoms
Decreased blood supply	(M) Impotence (F) Menstrual disorders
Decreased blood supply	Dryness and rashes
More energy immediately available	Rapid tiredness

its helpful abilities.[10] Later in this book suggestions aimed at increasing the ability to relax will be offered.

All of the body's 'rev-up' activity is designed to improve performance. But if the stress which launches this activity continues unabated, researchers believe, the human body begins to weaken as it is bombarded by stimulation and stress-related chemicals. Melhuish has described many of the long-term effects of pressure in Table 1.

As stress begins to take its toll on the body and mind, a variety of symptoms can result. Doctors have identified physical and mental symptoms of stress listed in Table 2 as commonly occurring before the onset of serious stress-related illness.

Doctors have also identified the ailments identified in Table 3 as having a stress background, meaning they may be brought on or aggravated by stress.

HYPERTENSION AND HEART DISEASE

Stress is seen to play a part in diseases related to lifestyle, where the degree to which a person eats, smokes, drinks alcohol and exercises plays a role. The first two illnesses in the list of ailments, high blood pressure and heart disease, are accepted now as having a proven link to stress. Hypertension, or raised blood pressure, in most cases has no direct organic basis – it simply sets in. A majority of cases are diagnosed as 'essential hypertension', meaning they don't arise from any medically correctable function.

Although other factors such as diet, obesity and smoking surely play a role, many researchers now believe stress is the primary cause of hypertension. The connection, as Andrew Melhuish indicates, is as follows: hypertension is believed to result partially from changes in the resistance of the blood vessels.[11] The tension of the arterial vessels, which carry blood to the tissues, is partly controlled by the sympathetic nervous system and its release of chemicals through the vessels. Continual activation of the sympathetic nervous system's chemical response is believed to result in reduced elasticity of the arteries and raised blood pressure. This resulting hypertension can lead to heart disease because of the increased

Table 2.

Physical Symptoms of Stress	Mental Symptoms of Stress
Lack of appetite	Constant irritability with people
Craving for food when under pressure	Feeling unable to cope
Frequent indigestion or heartburn	Lack of interest in life
Constipation or diarrhoea	Constant, or recurrent fear of disease
Insomnia	A feeling of being a failure
Constant tiredness	A feeling of being bad or of self-hatred
Tendency to sweat for no good reason	Difficulty in making decisions
Nervous twitches	A feeling of ugliness
Nail biting	Loss of interest in other people
Headaches	Awareness of suppressed anger
Cramps and muscle spasms	Inability to show true feelings
Nausea	A feeling of being the target of other people's animosity
Breathlessness without exertion	Loss of sense of humour
Fainting spells	Feeling of neglect
Frequent crying or desire to cry	Dread of the future
Impotency or frigidity	A feeling of having failed as a person or parent
Inability to sit still without fidgeting	A feeling of having no one to confide in
High blood pressure	Difficulty in concentrating
	The inability to finish one task before rushing on to the next
	An intense fear of open or enclosed spaces, or of being alone

Table 3. List of Ailments
Recognized to have Stress Background

Hypertension: high blood pressure	Rheumatoid arthritis
	Menstrual difficulties
Coronary thrombosis: heart attack	Nervous dyspepsia:
Migraine	flatulence and
Hay fever and allergies	indigestion
Asthma	Hyperthyroidism: overactive
Pruritus: intense itching	thyroid gland
Peptic ulcers	Diabetes mellitus
Constipation	Skin disorders
Colitis	Tuberculosis
	Depression

workload on the heart as it pushes blood out against a high arterial pressure. Also, high blood pressure increases the likelihood of a possibly fatal ruptured artery; the rupture of a vessel in the brain can cause stroke. Chronic stress, and its resulting release of fats into the bloodstream during the 'fight or flight' response, is also believed to increase the risk of coronary heart disease by adding fatty deposits to the lining of the coronary arteries, which provide oxygen to the heart muscle. Figure 3, 'Flight Path to a Heart Attack', shows the combination of factors that can result in a life-threatening crisis.[12]

CANCER

Some researchers are exploring the connection between stress and cancer, believing stress may cause a suppression of the immune system. Bernard H. Fox suggests there are two primary mechanisms causing cancer: first, 'carcinogenesis, the production of cancer by an agent or mechanism overcoming existing resistance of the body'; and second, 'lowered resistance to cancer, which permits a potential carcinogen normally insufficient to produce cancer, to do so'.[13] In addition, recent research has identified behavioural and stress related components in the onset of cancer. Although stress has by

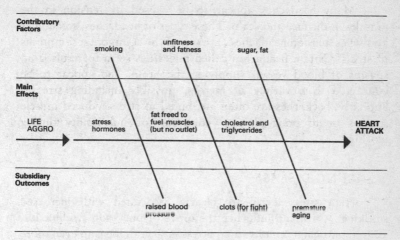

LIFE AGGRO refers to life 'aggravation': stress agents at work, in the home, etc.

Figure 3. Flight Path to a Heart Attack
Source: an adaptation from Malcolm Carruthers, Maudsley Hospital

no means been identified as playing a major role in the onset of cancer, a study of 2,000 women attending breast screening clinics found that a greater percentage of women who developed breast cancer had in the previous two years suffered a loss, such as the death of a husband, friend or relative, than had those with normal breasts.[14]

STOMACH AND INTESTINAL PROBLEMS

Certain individuals appear to respond to stress with an increase in the production of stomach acid, often contributing to ulcers of the stomach or duodenum (first part of the small intestine). Other conditions which are believed to be brought on or aggravated by chronic stress include ulcerative colitis, or bleeding ulcerations in the large intestine, and irritable bowel syndrome, which involves painful spasms in the large intestine.[15]

HEADACHES, BACKACHES

Many headaches appear to be caused by tension in the muscles in the face and scalp. These types of headaches, sometimes known as 'tension headaches', are one of the commonest symptoms of stress. Certain headaches called migraines seem to result from spasms of blood vessels supplying the brain, and appear to be connected to a variety of factors, possibly including stress.[16] Similarly, backaches are often attributed to stress-induced muscle spasms or to poor physical condition or inflexibility during working.

LUNG DISEASE

High stress levels are clearly associated with increased smoking, which can influence the onset of pneumonia, influenza, and, in particular, emphysema. Stress is seen to have an even more direct influence in precipitating asthma attacks. Asthma attacks are not ordinarily the result of a single cause, but in one widespread investigation, emotional factors were found to be present in 70 per cent of the asthmatic patients studied.[17]

SKIN PROBLEMS

Skin diseases are a highly visible consequence of the aggravating effects of stress. Eczema, hives, and acne are all skin conditions believed to be associated with stress. For example, one study demonstrated that 'in eczema-prone individuals, emotional arousal leads to specific changes in the skin cells'.[18]

The mental and physical health risks faced by each individual coping poorly with prolonged stress cannot be predicted exactly; it is clear, however, that the potential costs to the individual can be enormous. Before looking at how each person can analyse his or her own stress level and act to reduce it, we will take a closer look at the individual costs of stress and how they are magnified at organizational and national levels.

Chapter Two

THE COSTS OF STRESS

The World is too much with us; late and soon,
Getting and spending, we lay waste our powers.
William Wordsworth, 1807

To the individual whose health or happiness has been ravaged by the effects of stress, the costs involved are only too clear. Whether manifested as minor complaints of illness, serious ailments such as heart disease, or social problems such as alcoholism and drug abuse, stress-related problems exact a heavy payment. It has also long been recognized that a family suffers indirectly from the stress problems of one of its members – suffering that takes the form of unhappy marriages, divorces, and spouse and child abuse. But what price do organizations and nations pay for a poor fit between people and their environments? Only recently has stress been seen as contributing to the health costs of companies and countries. But as studies of stress-related illnesses and deaths show, stress is taking a devastatingly high toll on our combined productivity and health.

HEALTH COSTS: THE HIGH PRICE WE PAY

Chapter 1 explained how certain ailments are linked to stress, especially to prolonged chronic stress, and described how the leading killer – heart and circulatory disease – has been shown to have a connection with stress levels. Cancer, a second major cause of death, is increasingly being linked to lifestyle factors. The descriptions and figures below paint a gloomy picture of the extent to which these ailments, as well as other conditions, strike our family members, friends and fellow workers.

HEART AND CIRCULATORY DISEASES

Heart and blood vessel diseases have risen steadily during the past several decades. Between the 1950s and the 1970s in England and Wales the death rate for men aged 34 to 44 due to coronary heart disease nearly doubled. Notably, death rates for men in these prime working ages increased more rapidly than that of the older age ranges. By 1973, 41 per cent of all deaths in the age group 35 to 44 were due to cardiovascular disease, with nearly 30 per cent due to coronary heart disease. By the mid seventies, myocardial infarction (heart attack) was far and away the leading cause of death in men and had increased by 80 per cent over the previous 25 years, as shown in Table 1.

Diseases of the circulatory system combined to be the second largest reason for sickness and invalidity benefit in Great Britain between June 1976 and June 1977. Today in Britain, as a Health Education Council report noted, coronary heart disease remains the leading cause of death and 'kills more than 150,000 people each year – one person every three to four minutes. One man in eleven dies of a heart attack before he is sixty-five years old.'

Almost half of all Americans die of cardiovascular disease, which includes heart attack and stroke. The resulting economic cost, including medical services and lost productivity, reached an estimated \$78.6 billion in 1986. Heart attack is the leading cause of death in the USA, followed by cancer and stroke.[2] It is also estimated that more than \$700 million a year is spent by American employers to replace the 200,000 men aged 45 to 65 who die or are incapacitated by coronary heart disease.[3]

However, the United States has succeeded in reversing the long prevailing upward trend in heart and vascular diseases. As Table 2 shows, between 1968 and 1977, deaths of American men due to ischaemic heart disease fell 27 per cent, while in England and Wales, male deaths increased 3 per cent. Correspondingly, deaths of American women dropped 31 per cent, while deaths of women in England and Wales increased by 11 per cent between 1968 and 1977. (Table 3 shows a ranking order of deaths due to heart disease by countries during the same period.)

Table 1. Top 20 Causes of Deaths of Men in England and Wales in 1976

		Death rate per million population
1	Acute myocardial infarction	2,678
2	Cerebrovascular disease	1,200
3	Cancer of trachea, bronchus and lung	1,110
4	Myocardial degeneration	1,051
5	Pneumonia	994
6	Bronchitis	717
7	Cancer of stomach	289
8	Cancer of prostate	192
9	Cancer of large intestine (except rectum)	186
10	Motor vehicle traffic accidents	171
11	Aortic aneurysm (non-syphilitic)	152
12	Hypertensive disease	142
13	Cancer of rectum	139
14	Arteriosclerosis	138
15	Cancer of bladder	123
16	Cancer of pancreas	119
17	Influenza	106
18	Suicide	97
19	Chronic rheumatic heart disease	87
20	Diabetes mellitus	86
	Total deaths in 1976	12,527

Source: OPCS Mortality Statistics DH2

Table 2. Average Increase/Decrease in Mortality From Ischaemic Heart Disease 1968–77 (40–69 Age Group)

Men	% Decrease		% Increase
USA	27	Scotland	1
Japan	25	England and Wales	3
Austria	20	Northern Ireland	12
Finland	18	Ireland	30
Norway	11	Hungary	
Holland	10	Poland	
Italy	2	Rumania	Over 30
		Bulgaria	
		Yugoslavia	

Women			
Japan	39	Scotland	10
USA	31	England and Wales	11
Italy	20	Hungary	
Finland	15	Poland	
France	14	Rumania	Over 20
Norway	2	Bulgaria	
Northern Ireland	0	Yugoslavia	

Source: WHO, *World Health Statistics* 35 (1), 1982.

Between 1972 and 1983, the annual American death rate due to coronary heart disease fell a total of 31 per cent, and deaths due to stroke fell 47 per cent.[4] Some research indicates this positive trend can be partly attributed to lifestyle changes in the US such as

Table 3. Heart Disease Deaths per 100,000 (40–69 Age Group)

Women		Men	
Scotland	202	Finland	673
Israel	193	Scotland	615
Northern Ireland	189	Northern Ireland	614
USA	171	USA	528
Ireland	168	Ireland	508
Finland	142	England and Wales	498
England and Wales	138	West Germany	325
Bulgaria	110	Bulgaria	237
West Germany	84	Poland	229
Italy	63	France	152
France	37	Japan	69
Japan	29		

Source: WHO, *World Health Statistics*, 35 (1), 1982.

increased exercise, altered diet and reduced smoking. Efforts are under way in Britain and European countries to reproduce this improvement.

In Britain, coronary heart disease is generally twice as prevalent in men as in women, but the disease's rate of increase over the years has been even greater in women. Furthermore, as Table 4 shows, days lost from work by British women between 1982–3 and 1984–5 increased dramatically due to causes of heart disease and cerebrovascular disease over a two-year period.

Heart disease increased as a cause for lost days by more than 25 per cent for women (as compared to 13 per cent for men) and cerebrovascular disease increased by more than 73 per cent for women (as compared to more than 12 per cent for men). In the US, where deaths due to heart disease have been declining for both

Table 4. Days Lost in Britain From Work for Certain Mental and Stress-related Causes

Cause	Male/Female	1982/3	1984/5	% Change over two years
Psychoses	M	7,098,538	8,138,000	+16.04
	F	3,253,344	3,275,080	+ 0.66
Neuroses	M	17,432,981	17,938,743	+ 2.90
	F	9,951,749	10,162,450	+ 2.18
Personality disorders	M	160,100	162,200	+ 1.31
	F	153,600	131,600	−14.32
Mental retardation	M	1,312,400	1,310,286	− 0.17
	F	786,000	823,300	+ 4.74
Migraine	M	158,529	136,300	−14.02
	F	177,683	62,800	−64.65
Hypertensive diseases	M	9,477,164	9,890,527	+ 4.36
	F	1,997,336	2,060,400	+ 3.16
Ulcers	M	2,216,132	2,088,828	− 1.75
	F	294,295	312,659	+ 6.24
Depressive disorder	M	6,439,698	6,134,613	− 4.47
	F	4,276,919	4,201,100	− 1.77
Alcohol dependence	M	896,600	895,401	− 0.13
	F	79,600	38,800	−51.26
Ischaemic heart disease	M	29,092,909	32,912,455	+13.13
	F	1,908,911	2,389,044	+25.15
Cerebro-vascular disease	M	6,222,500	7,011,600	+12.68
	F	529,800	920,700	+73.78
Total days lost in above causes	M	80,417,551	86,618,953	+ 7.71
	F	23,409,237	24,377,933	+ 4.14
Total number of days lost	M	271,715,438	253,562,397	− 6.68
	F	89,229,711	74,546,812	−16.52

Source: Department of Health and Social Security (DHSS) tables, S/IV, *Employment Gazette*, August 1986.

sexes, death rates due to coronary heart disease for men aged 35–64 fell 14.2 per cent between 1979 and 1983, but fell only 7.7 per cent for women of the same ages. As will be discussed in Chapter 4, studies are providing some interesting clues as to how recent changes in women's roles are affecting their overall mental and physical health.

Stroke is the third leading cause of death among adult Americans, resulting in 156,400 deaths in 1983.[5] The connection between coping poorly with stress and the development of strokes and related circulatory diseases is believed similar to the relationship between stress and heart attack.

Another disease increasingly linked to stress is high blood pressure (hypertension). In 1983, it was estimated that nearly 55 million adult Americans – nearly one in every four – suffered from hypertension.[6] Hypertension, like heart disease and cerebrovascular disease, has increased as a cause of absence from work in Britain between 1982–3 and 1984–5 (see Table 4).

CANCER

Recent research has identified behavioural and stress-related components in the onset of cancer, as we discussed in Chapter 1. Recent evidence suggests that in both the US and Britain, overall cancer incidence and death rates have been steadily increasing. Research from the American Cancer Society shows a significant rise in cancer deaths in England and Wales between 1970–71 and 1980–81. In 1970–71, an average of 186 men per 100,000 population died of cancer. Ten years later, 244 men per 100,000 died of cancer, a 31 per cent increase. During the same decade, female cancer deaths grew from 119 to 157 per 100,000 population, a 32 per cent rise.

Deaths due to lung cancer during the decade grew substantially for British men and startlingly for British women. Male deaths due to lung cancer grew from 72 to 93 per 100,000 population, a 28 per cent increase. While this jump is serious enough, the picture becomes alarming for British women: the lung cancer death rate grew from 12 deaths to 22 deaths per 100,000 population, a 77 per cent increase.

England and Wales rank first among forty-seven countries in the death rate of women due to breast cancer. Between 1970–71 and 1980–81, the rate grew from 26 to 34 per 100,000, a 30 per cent rise. In contrast, there was only a slight (2 per cent) increase in uterine cancer deaths.

The US ranks above mid-point in most cancer categories. Overall, male cancer deaths per 100,000 grew 38 per cent between 1970–71 and 1980–81. Deaths of American women grew 27 per cent during the same period. Once again, the most dramatic jump in deaths occurred for women dying of lung cancer. During the decade, female deaths per 100,000 population grew from 9.4 to 21.4, a 128 per cent increase!

SMOKING: THE LINK TO HEART DISEASE AND CANCER

People commonly turn to tobacco as a means to deal with stressful situations, studies show. For example, one investigation of 35,000 nurses in the UK found that smoking was one of the most commonly identified ways of coping with stress.[7] The price smokers pay is high. As the American Heart Association notes, 'cigarette smoking is the biggest risk factor for sudden cardiac death: smokers have between two to four times the risk of non-smokers'.[8] As physician Andrew Melhuish points out, 'some 30 major studies in 10 countries have drawn an inescapable correlation between smoking and lung cancer: the heavy smoker is 20 times more likely to contract this dreadful disease than the non-smoker.'[9]

Cigarette smoking is believed to be responsible for 85 per cent of lung cancer cases among men and 75 per cent among women. In the US, smoking contributes to an estimated 350,000 premature deaths each year.[10] The cost of smoking to the US economy has been estimated at about $65 billion due to lost productivity and medical treatment for smoking-related diseases.[11] High smoking levels are associated with neurosis and anxiety as well as physical illness.[12]

On a more positive note, smoking rates are declining. Between 1945 and 1972 smoking rates remained steady for men and increased in women. But smoking rates fell dramatically in Britain between 1972 and 1982, leaving smokers as a minority. In 1972, 53 per cent of all men were smokers, while only 38 per cent of men smoked by 1982. Within the same decade, the percentage of women smoking fell from 41 per cent to 33 per cent.[13] Between 1976 and 1985, male smokers in the US dropped from 42 per cent of the population to 33 per cent, while women smokers declined from 32 per cent to 28 per cent.[14] The relatively smaller decrease in smoking among women may relate to an increased search for coping mechanisms among women juggling stressful home and work situations.

WHO SUFFERS MOST – THE SURPRISING ANSWER

It is commonly believed that executives and other white-collar workers suffer the most from stress-related illnesses. Intense office situations with demanding deadlines, the required attention to detail and complex interpersonal relations are often believed to produce high levels of stress and strain.

Yet, as Table 5 shows, the frequencies of deaths due to major causes in the working population increase as we move from professional and white-collar jobs down to the unskilled. This applies both to stress-related illnesses such as ischaemic heart disease and to other illnesses such as pneumonia and prostate cancer. These statistics are very similar to those of US workers. This pattern extends not only to deaths but to illnesses as well. It can be seen in Table 6 that many blue-collar workers show a greater number of restricted activity days and consultations with general practitioners than do white-collar workers in the UK.

MENTAL ILLNESS*

The breakdown of an individual's mental health has been increasingly linked by medics and stress researchers to the level of life stress he or she experiences. Although we will discuss ab-

---

* Some of the material from this section comes from NIOSH's proposed *National Strategy on the Prevention of Work-related Psychological Disorders*, October 1986.

Table 5. UK Deaths due to Major Causes and Types of Occupations, 1970–72 (standardized mortality rates = 100)*

Causes of deaths, persons aged 15–64 (males)	Professional and similar	Intermediate
Trachea, bronchus, and lung cancer	53	68
Prostate cancer	91	89
Ischaemic heart disease	88	91
Other forms of heart disease	69	75
Cerebrovascular disease	80	86
Pneumonia	41	53
Bronchitis, emphysema and asthma	36	51
All causes	77	81

*100 represents the average number of deaths in each category in the population as a whole. For example, professionals are about half as likely to die from trachea, bronchus, and lung cancer as is the average person.

Source: UK Office of Population Censuses and Surveys

senteeism in more detail later in this chapter, a look at work lost due to mental health problems indicates the magnitude of the problem. Of the 328 million days lost from work in Britain in 1984–5, 53 million, or 16 per cent, were due to mental health causes, as can be seen in Table 4. A look at the reasons given by British men for days off due to stress-related illness (Table 7) shows a huge increase over a twenty-five-year period in the category of 'nervousness, debility and headache'.

In one effort to determine how widespread mental health problems are in the US, 17,000 people were interviewed at five regional sites as part of a government study. Results showed that over a six-month period, between 17 and 23 per cent of those interviewed had experienced at least one major psychological disorder. Between 7 to 15 per cent reported having had at least one anxiety disorder. When questioned about a lifetime's incidence of

Skilled, non-manual	Skilled manual	Partly skilled	Unskilled
84	118	123	143
99	115	106	115
114	107	108	111
94	100	121	157
98	106	111	136
78	92	115	195
82	113	128	188
99	106	114	137

mental health problems, between 29 and 38 per cent said they had suffered one or more major disorders. As the government study stated, 'psychological disorders were most common during the prime working ages of 25 to 44 years'.[15]

A separate study in the late 1970s of those receiving Social Security disability allowances in the US showed that mental disorders were the third most disabling condition, and they represented 11 per cent of all disability allowances.[16]

In 1980, 150 top female managers in the UK were questioned about their overall psychological and physical ill health. Table 8 shows the percentage of women who reported having stress-related physical and psychological symptoms of illness. It is interesting to see that with the exception of migraine headaches, few physical problems were reported; however, a high percentage reported having experienced psychological problems, with irritation, anxiety and tiredness being experienced by well over half of the women.

Table 6. Acute Sickness and Consultations with U K General Medical Practitioners, 1974–5

	Average number of restricted activity days per person per year (males)			Average number of consultations per person per year (males)		
	15–44	45–64	All ages	15–44	45–64	All ages
Professional	9	16	12	2.1	2.7	2.7
Employers and managers	11	13	14	1.8	2.4	2.7
Intermediate and junior non-manual	10	21	15	2.0	4.3	3.1
Skilled manual and own account non-professional	15	24	17	2.8	4.0	3.2
Semi-skilled manual and personal service	16	23	18	2.7	4.5	3.7
Unskilled, manual	21	28	20	3.5	4.8	3.6
All persons	13	21	16	2.4	3.8	3.1

Source: *General Household Survey*, 1974 and 1975

Other evidence of the mental suffering being experienced:

- It has been found that the relaxant Valium is the fourth most commonly prescribed drug for Americans.[17] In 1984, psychotherapeutic drugs made up approximately 25 per cent of all out-patient prescriptions.[18]
- In Britain, 5 per cent of men and 12 per cent of women were on tranquillizers in 1976. By the mid 1970s the number of prescriptions for tranquillizers dispensed by the National Health Service in England had grown significantly (Table 9).[19]
- Health costs for mental illness are reported to exceed $36 billion each year in the US.[20]

- A recent survey showed that 3.3 per cent of all visits to US internists resulted in diagnosis of mental illness. For individuals between 25 and 44 years of age, the percentage was nearly double.[21]
- In England, general practice consultation rates for mental disorders were 300 per 1,000 population, exceeded only by coughs, colds and bronchitis (Table 10).[22]
- A recent study of general practice surgeries in the US showed patients' most common complaints during visitation involved psychological problems.[23]
- A study of a large out-patient and hospital care organization in the Washington, D.C. area found that 'anxiety/stress' was the topic most demanded by their patients in terms of health education and promotion.[24]

Mental health problems have long been associated with various occupations. As the NIOSH report suggests, 'mental disturbances, especially severe mental illnesses, are most heavily concentrated among workers with lower income, lower education, less skilled and less prestigious jobs'.[25]

Table 7. Percentage Increase in Absenteeism From 1954–5 to 1978–9 Due to Stress-related Illness (Men Only)

Diagnosis	Increase %
Nervousness, debility, headache	528
Ill-defined symptoms	101
Psychoneuroses and psychoses	49
Heart disease	134
Other forms of heart disease	38
Hypertensive disease	123

Source: Peter Hingley and Cary Cooper, *Stress and the Nurse Manager*, 1986.

Table 8. Women Managers Reporting Physical and Psychological Illness

Physical	%	Psychological	%
Gastric and/or peptic ulcer	4.4	Anger	35.6
Asthma	2.2	Irritation	60.0
High blood pressure	9.6	Anxiety	50.4
Migraine headaches	27.4	Tiredness	69.6
Eczema	5.9	Low self-esteem	25.9
Heart disease	0	Depression	23.7
Arthritis and/or rheumatoid arthritis	8.1	Tension (neck or back)	42.2
Stroke	0	Sleeplessness	34.1
		Frustration	34.8
		Dissatisfaction with life or job	34.1

Source: C. L. Cooper, *Executive Families Under Stress*, 1982.

ALCOHOL ABUSE

'Turning to drink' is a coping mechanism adopted by all too many of us, according to studies. Between 1 and 5 per cent of the British population are estimated to suffer from drinking problems.[26] According to stress researcher Hans Selye, high levels of drinking are clearly more common in stressful occupations.[27] A study mentioned earlier of more than 35,000 nurses in the UK found that alcohol, smoking and caffeine were the most common ways of dealing with stress. The idea that alcohol consumption is related to job stress is bolstered by looking at a separate study of the drinking levels of nurse managers as compared to that of women in general. While national figures indicate that 4.8 per cent of the female population drinks daily, the incidence of daily drinking among nurse managers was nearly double at 8 per cent.[28]

Table 9. N H S Prescriptions (in Millions) for Tranquillizers Dispensed in England and Wales

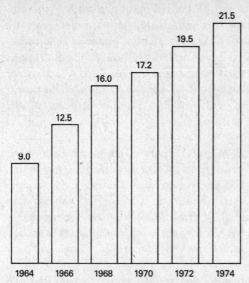

Source: A. Melhuish, *Executive Health*, 1978

Table 10. General Practice Consultation Rates for Specific Illnesses

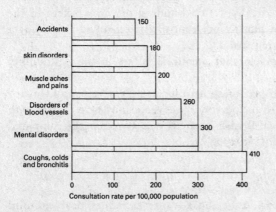

Source: A. Melhuish, *Executive Health*, 1978

Problems associated with heavy drinking include 'the loss of jobs, cirrhosis of the liver, suicide, marriage breakdown, child abuse and accidents at home or work', according to one study.[29] In addition to the personal havoc this can create, the economic costs are staggering. A look at alcoholism and alcohol abuse in 1980 estimated the costs to the US economy at $89.5 billion. Problem drinkers were found to be more than 20 per cent less productive than other workers, a situation which accounted for $49.8 billion of the cost.[30]

Studies of drinking problems in a number of occupational groups have shown the following:

- Of 500 commercial airline pilots interviewed, 99 per cent are at least occasional drinkers of alcohol. On days they are not flying, they said they consumed an average of five drinks a day. 13 per cent indicated they used alcohol as a means of coping with stress. 52 per cent said they drink more than two drinks a day and 13 per cent have been told they drink too much. More than a quarter of the pilots felt they needed to cut down on their drinking.[31]
- In another occupation involving serious safety factors, the offshore oil and gas industry, there seems to be a strong link between stress, alcohol consumption and accidents. As Robert Burke, editor of *Offshore*, suggests, 'one aspect of safety not discussed in polite places is the use and abuse of drugs and alcohol on a rig'.[32] In fact, a study of about two hundred oil rig workers in the North Sea found that 61 per cent often consumed alcohol as a method of relieving stress.
- It has been estimated that alcoholic nurses in the US number 40,000.[33]
- Alcohol abuse is becoming an increasingly severe problem for women. In 1980–81, 1 person in 2.4 requesting help to deal with alcoholism at local British councils was a woman, as compared to 1 in 4 applicants in 1974.[34]

DRUG ABUSE

Like alcoholism, drug abuse is often a hidden problem until it becomes impossible to hide. It has been estimated, however, that the chemically addicted employee is almost four times as likely to be involved in an accident, 'receives three times the average level of sick benefits', and is 'five times as likely to file a worker's compensation claim'.[35] In the US, decreased productivity due to drug abuse has been estimated at $26 billion a year.[36]

COSTS IN THE WORKPLACE

All of the potential stress costs outlined in this chapter combine both to lessen the satisfaction obtained from work and reduce on-the-job performance. Chapter 4 will look more closely at how work influences stress levels, but it is relevant here to mention the ways in which stress is reflected in the workplace.

JOB SATISFACTION

At least one study shows that job satisfaction among US workers fell during the 1970s.[37] The US experience was reinforced in other industrialized countries. For example, between a quarter and a third of Swedish workers described their work as often 'stressful'.[38]

Stress levels in various occupations are known to differ. Certain occupations, such as mining, piloting, police work, advertising and acting are believed to provide the highest stress levels.

Stress on the job becomes an occupational hazard for certain 'helping' professionals, such as physicians, dentists, nurses, and health technologists, who 'have higher than expected rates of suicide and alcohol/drug abuse'.[39] 'Burnout', or the premature retirement from one's career due to stress, appears particularly common among nurses. Nurses and others in the health field suffer from mental ill health to the extent that more of them are being admitted to hospitals and clinics for the treatment of mental disorders than in previous years.[40]

JOB PERFORMANCE

It has been proved in experiments and studies that, within certain limits, an individual's performance actually improves with

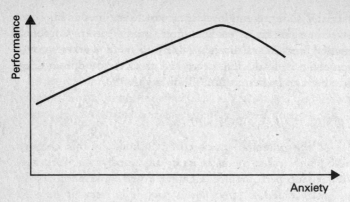

Figure 1. Effect of Anxiety on Performance: Yerkes-Dodson Law
Source: A. Melhuish, *Executive Health*, 1978

increased levels of stress. After a point, however, stress clearly results in reduced performance. The Yerkes-Dodson law, as shown in Figure 1, resulted from experiments which measured the performance of mice at different levels of anxiety. Figure 2 interprets this phenomenon in medical terms. 'The portion of the graph

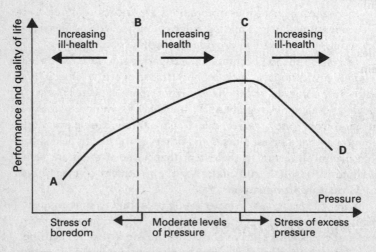

Figure 2. Medical Extension of Yerkes-Dodson Law
Source: A. Melhuish, *Executive Health*, 1978

between B and C represents pressures which the individual can tolerate: within these limits his health and quality of life improve with increased pressure (challenge). At C, however, increased pressure loses its beneficial effect and becomes harmful. Pressure becomes stress and in the portion C–D, health and quality of life decrease. C is the threshold (as is B, for boredom is also a potent stress and the portion B–A also represents increasing risk of stress illness).'[41]

ABSENTEEISM AND TURNOVER OF LABOUR FORCE

Absenteeism is one of the most obvious costs of stress to employers. In general, indications are that absenteeism is a widespread and accelerating problem in many occupations. By the 1970s, it was recognized that time lost from work due to stress-related illnesses cost Britain far more than losses due to work stoppages and strikes. In 1970 the Confederation of British Industry reported that absenteeism 'has risen alarmingly in recent years in spite of improvements in social and working conditions, income levels, and family health'.[42] In 1984–5, 328 million days of work were lost in Great Britain (Table 5). In at least one occupation, nursing, short-term absences among nurses are increasingly being blamed on clinical anxiety and depression believed to result from occupational strain.[43]

High rates of employee turnover can become quite expensive to a company – they raise training costs, reduce overall efficiency and disrupt other workers. Although it is hard to estimate the actual costs of labour turnover, it is thought that they often equal about five times an employee's monthly salary.[44]

Costs to a Company

Karl Albrecht, an American organizational development consultant, has estimated the cost of stress to a hypothetical firm of 2,000 employees with sales of about $60 million a year.[45] Focusing primarily on costs historically due to absenteeism and staff turnover, he makes the following estimate:

Firm size: 2,000 people

Sales: $60 million a year

Profit: 5 per cent, or $3 million a year

Average salary (gross average for all employees): $6.00 an hour

Personnel costs (salary and overhead) per day: $100 a person

Absentee rate (excluding vacation): 4 per cent = 10 days per person per year

Turnover rate (assume stable size of work-force) per year: 5 per cent = 100 people per year

Stress-linked absenteeism: $1,000,000 a year

Stress-linked turnover: $40,000 a year

Company performance degradation (overstaffing cost): $2,500,000 a year

Antisocial acts: $20,000 a year

TOTAL $3,560,000 a year

LITIGATION AND HEALTH CARE COSTS

Employers are paying directly for stress-related illnesses through workers' compensation claims. 'In general, claims for psychological disorders suffered as the result of job experiences have multiplied over the decade of the '70s . . . in 1979, the State of California alone received more than 3,000–4,000 "psychiatric" injury claims, half of which resulted in monetary awards.'[46] J. M. Ivancevich and his colleagues at the University of Houston have recently reviewed three landmark court cases which have resulted in American corporations increasingly being held responsible for workplace stress.[47] In 1955, an iron worker named Bailey saw a fellow scaffolding worker fall to his death. Bailey returned to work, but gradually he began to have frequent black-outs and became paralysed. He also suffered from sleeping difficulties and extreme sensitivity to pain. In the resulting court case, *Bailey* v. *American General*, a Texas court ruled in Bailey's favour. The physical accident and psychological trauma were held responsible for the onset of the subsequent paralysis and other problems. Although not a radical decision, it paved the way for compensation cases under existing laws. In a dramatic case in 1960, the Michigan Supreme Court ruled that an assembly worker's psychological breakdown might have been due not only to the difficulty of keeping up with his machine-paced work, but also to his supervisor's repeated criticisms of his performance. In this case, *Carter* v. *General Motors*, a broader interpretation was made of America's workers' compensation laws, which state the workers must be compensated 'for all work-related injuries'. In the past, only a 'discrete, identifiable accident' could be compensated for. In this case, the 'cumulative trauma' that Carter suffered over a long period was held responsible for his breakdown. The third landmark case, *Alcorn* v. *Arbo Engineering*, involved a lorry driver named Alcorn who was in disagreement with management over his union activities. Alcorn claimed that abusive behaviour by his managers had led to physical and emotional distress and that he suffered from insomnia, nausea and other symptoms. In a 1970 ruling, Alcorn won his compensation claim. These three cases described are now established in American law in more than a dozen states and are used as precedents in many others. Many employers are being held responsible due to the belief that they are doing little to cut down the stressful aspects of many jobs. This may help to explain the growth in corporate health and stress management programmes in America. Those employers who are at least seen to be doing something about workplace stress may be able to put forward a better defence in the courts.

According to a US government report, one specific type of compensation claim, 'gradual mental stress', has shown significant growth in recent years. As the report explains, this type of claim refers to 'cumulative emotional problems stemming mainly from exposure to adverse psychosocial conditions at work . . . Emotional problems related to a specific traumatic event at work, or to work-related physical disease or injury, such as witnessing a severe accident, are not included'. According to the report, about 11 per cent of all occupational disease claims involve gradual mental stress. In addition, 'worker compensation costs for gradual mental stress reached and then surpassed average costs for other occupational disease claims in the period 1981–1982'.[48]

LOSS OF VITALITY

Psychologists Jonathan Quick and James Quick have outlined a number of *indirect costs* which can result from mismanaged stress within an organization. As described below, these costs primarily involve loss of vitality, communication breakdown and faulty decision-making.[49]

It has been theorized that people have a certain level of 'superficial adaptive energy' which allows them to cope with stressful situations. When a person's stress level is 'at boiling point', and for a long period of time, his or her energy supply is so depleted that there is a 'limited bounce-back' or recuperative effect. Employees whose jobs do not allow them to maintain their energy reserves may eventually perform less well and contribute less to their organizations. As Quick and Quick suggest loss of vitality may result in low morale, low motivation and high dissatisfaction; and these indirect costs may contribute to direct costs of high staff turnover and low productivity.

MISCOMMUNICATION

When employees are experiencing high stress levels, communication breakdowns can result. The frequency with which employees communicate with each other has been shown to decline when there is a large degree of role conflict present. Role conflict, which will be discussed in Chapter 4, occurs when a person tries to meet two or more conflicting sets of expectations. The individuals experiencing the conflict tend to withdraw from the relationships causing them difficulty. High organizational stress levels also can result in communication distortion because employees under stress often feel defensive and may misinterpret messages they receive.

POOR DECISION-MAKING

When communication breakdowns occur, information may be lost or not conveyed, resulting in decisions being based upon incomplete or incorrect information. In addition, a decision-maker's judgement may be impaired during times of chronic stress.

An employee who is bored or under-utilized at work will be less decisive and responsive, while one suffering from work overload will be less rational and unable to explore all the alternatives available.

The individual costs of stress, as they cumulate within families, organizations and countries, add up to a major cause of lost happiness, productivity and potential achievement. Just as damage from stress first affects an individual, so can the process of learning to cope with stress begin at the individual level. This process often begins with a person's recognition of his or her own personality traits and how they translate into individual coping styles, as will be discussed in Chapter 3.

Chapter Three

THE INDIVIDUAL AND STRESS

'We boil at different degrees.'
Ralph Waldo Emerson, 1870

Life hands each of us a measure of strain, pressure and misfortune. And while some individuals may appear to have an undue share of problems and calamities, nearly everyone is confronted daily with potentially stressful situations. It is the individual's repeated response to these situations which can snowball into chronic stress levels. Why, we can wonder, are certain individuals more vulnerable than others to the stress agents they encounter? Extensive study of the stress response has led researchers to identify some key factors that influence an individual's vulnerability to stress. Primarily, the individual's personality, coping strategies, and the number and nature of events encountered are seen to vitally affect stress vulnerability. In addition, certain characteristics of age, sex, and ethnic background, as well as the degree of social support each person receives, have emerged as indicators of vulnerability.

PERSONALITY

Consider a number of individuals waiting for service at a bank teller's window. Jack's impatience is clear: he shuffles his feet, strains to see what is happening ahead of him, sighs in exasperation and aims angry looks at the clerk. In contrast, Susan would appear the epitome of patience and calm as she waits, her face composed, a slight smile upon her lips. But a sharp observer would detect the tightening of her jaw and the tic at the corner of one eye as Susan attempts to conceal her anger. Both Jack and

Susan may be paying an emotional and even physical toll as they wait. Their reactions, though different, are both totally unlike that of Mark, who is truly unconcerned about the wait. He gazes out of the bank window, interested in the flow of life on the street, enjoying the chance of pause for a moment. Just behind him, Tracey is using the time to jot down a shopping list and plan what she will cook for dinner.

The personalities and resultant coping styles of the four people described above act together to determine whether the same situation induces a stress response in each. For example, both Jack and Susan are experiencing varying levels of anxiety and distress as they wait, and furthermore, neither has found a coping style to relieve this reaction. Mark's relaxed personality is naturally such that he has no need to adjust to the situation, while Tracey, who, like Jack and Susan, can find waiting stressful, has learned to cope by occupying herself with a useful task which makes her feel more in control of her time.

Through studies and experiments, researchers have identified personality 'types' which appear to be more 'stress prone' than other individuals. In this and the following section, we will consider those behavioural factors and coping styles which can lead to high stress levels or exacerbate stress-related illness.

TYPE A: CORONARY-PRONE PERSONALITY

One of the most important research approaches to individual stress differences began in the early 1960s, when two researchers, Meyer Friedman and Ray Rosenman, developed a susceptibility profile to coronary heart disease.[2] It was found that the coronary patients under study behaved similarly in many ways – they were extremely competitive, high-achieving, aggressive, hasty, impatient and restless. They were characterized by explosive speech patterns, tenseness of facial muscles, and appearing to be under pressure of time and the challenge of responsibility. These individuals were described as 'Type A' personality types, as opposed to the more relaxed 'Type B', who had a low risk of coronary heart disease. One researcher noted of Type As in 1971 that 'people having this particular behavioural pattern were often deeply involved and committed to their work so that other aspects of their lives were relatively neglected'.[3]

A study (the Western Collaborative Group Study) of more than 3,400 American men in the mid 1960s did much to confirm the relationship between coronary heart disease and Type A behaviour. All of the men, who were free of coronary disease at the start of the study, were evaluated by psychiatrists through extensive interviews as being Type A or Type B. The psychiatrists were not provided with any biological data about the patients. Two and a half years after the evaluations, the patients received medical examinations by independent medical internists who were not aware of behavioural classifications. It was found that Type A men between the ages of 39 and 49 had 6.5 times the incidence of coronary heart disease as did the Type B men. Type A men between the ages of 50 and 59 had 1.9 times the incidence of coronary heart disease as did their Type B contemporaries. The Type A men also had a number of symptoms or risk factors of heart disease such as high blood pressure and high cholesterol levels. After four and a half years of study, the same relationship between behavioural types and coronary heart disease was found, with the Type A men having significantly higher incidence of different forms of heart disease.[4]

Over the years, other researchers have attempted to see if there is indeed a link between Type A behaviour and stress indicators. For example, a University of Michigan study in the mid 1970s contradicted the earlier results, saying that no significant correlations were found between Type A behaviour and various stress measures such as job dissatisfaction, sleeping disorders, anxiety, depression, irritation and physical stress. The researchers found instead that Type A behaviour acted as an intervening factor: when Type A behaviour was combined with work and family stress factors it predicted stress-related illness.[5] Other studies have indicated that Type A behaviour may lie dormant until the individual is faced with a challenging stressful situation; at that time, the combination of Type A behaviour and an extensive stress agent may trigger a physical reaction such as a heart attack. Still other studies have shown that Type A individuals may have higher blood pressure and cholesterol levels, and be inclined to smoke more and exercise less than their Type B counterparts, increasing their susceptibility to coronary heart disease.[6]

In addition, a link between high-status jobs and Type A behaviour has been indicated. One study looked at 943 white-collar, middle-class males in Buffalo, New York. The men came from five different work settings: the administrative staff and professional staff of a state health agency, supervisory personnel from a public service organization, officers from industrial and trade unions, faculty at a major private university and administrative officers of a large banking corporation. 'Not only was the Type A behaviour pattern significantly related to status as measured by rank, level of occupational prestige and income, it was also found to be significantly related to rapid career achievement as indicated by rank and income relative to age.'[7]

A review of a number of studies bore out the connection between Type A personality and high occupational status and it was found that 'Type As tended to describe their jobs as having more responsibility, longer hours and heavier workloads than do Type Bs. Despite these factors, Type As in general did not report more job dissatisfaction, anxiety, or depression than do Type Bs.'[8]

IDENTIFYING TYPE A BEHAVIOUR

The original Type A theorists, M. D. Friedman and R. H. Rosenman, identified Type A characteristics in their book, *Type A Behaviour and Your Heart*. They outline the following characteristics of a Type A personality:

- 'Possessing the habit of explosively accentuating various key words in ordinary speech without real need and tending to utter the last few words of sentences far more rapidly than the opening words.' Friedman and Rosenman believe the first habit reflects underlying aggression or hostility while the second 'mirrors your underlying impatience with spending even the time required for your own (Type As') speech'.
- 'Always moving, walking and eating rapidly.'
- Feeling or revealing to others an 'impatience with the rate at which most events take place'. Finding it 'difficult to restrain

from hurrying the speech of others and resorting to the device of saying very quickly, over and over again, "uh huh, uh huh," or "yes yes, yes yes" to someone who is talking', urging him to hurry up. Often finishing the sentences of persons speaking.

- Often attempting to do two or more things at the same time, such as thinking about an irrelevant subject when listening to someone else speak. 'Similarly, [you can be identified as Type A] if while golfing or fishing you continue to ponder business or professional problems or while using an electric razor you attempt also to eat your breakfast or drive your car or if while driving your car you attempt to dictate letters for your secretary.' Rosenman and Friedman describe this 'polyphasic' activity as one of the most common traits of the Type A individual.

- Finding it always difficult to refrain from talking about or turning any conversation to themes which have personal interest. At times when this manoeuvre fails, pretending to listen but really remaining preoccupied with these personal thoughts.

- Almost always feeling vaguely guilty when attempting to relax or do nothing for even just a few hours.

- No longer noticing the more interesting or lovely things encountered during the day.

- Not having 'any time to spare to become the things worth being because you are so preoccupied with getting the things worth having'.

- Attempting to 'schedule more and more in less and less time'. Making fewer allowances for unforeseen events which might disrupt the schedule. Also having a 'chronic sense of time urgency' – a core aspect of the Type A personality.

- 'On meeting another severely afflicted Type A person, instead of feeling compassion for his affliction you find yourself compelled to "challenge" him. This is a tell-tale trait because no one arouses the aggressive, hostile feelings of one Type A subject more quickly than another Type A subject.'

- Resorting to 'certain characteristic gestures or nervous tics', such as clenching fists, or banging a hand upon a table for emphasis.

- Becoming increasingly committed to translating and evaluating personal activities and the activities of others in terms of 'numbers'.

Rosenman and Friedman also outline the following characteristics as indicating the Type B personality:

- Being 'completely free of all of the habits and exhibiting none of the traits of the Type A personality'.
- Never suffering from time urgency and impatience.
- Harbouring no 'free-floating hostility' and feeling no need to impress others with your achievements or accomplishments unless the situation demands.
- Playing in order to find relaxation and fun, not to demonstrate achievement at any cost.
- Being able to work without agitation, 'relax without guilt'.[9]

Type A Questionnaire

The authors of this book have developed a simple questionnaire based upon the work of R. W. Bortner[10] which can give an idea of the extent of an individual's Type A behaviour. Although more sophisticated measures exist, this questionnaire will give a rough idea of the degree to which Type A behaviour is present. Ways to manage this behaviour will be discussed in Chapter 7.

Table 1. Type A Behaviour

Circle one number for each of the statements below which best reflects the way you behave in your everyday life. For example, if you are generally on time for appointments, for the first point you would circle a number between 7 and 11. If you are usually casual about appointments you would circle one of the lower numbers between 1 and 5.

Casual about appointments	1 2 3 4 5 6 7 8 9 10 11	Never late
Not competitive	1 2 3 4 5 6 7 8 9 10 11	Very competitive
Good listener	1 2 3 4 5 6 7 8 9 10 11	Anticipates what others are going to say (nods, attempts to finish for them)
Never feels rushed (even under pressure)	1 2 3 4 5 6 7 8 9 10 11	Always rushed

Can wait patiently	1 2 3 4 5 6 7 8 9 10 11	Impatient while waiting
Takes things one at a time	1 2 3 4 5 6 7 8 9 10 11	Tries to do many things at once, thinks about what will do next
Slow deliberate talker	1 2 3 4 5 6 7 8 9 10 11	Emphatic in speech fast and forceful
Cares about satisfying him/herself no matter what others may think	1 2 3 4 5 6 7 8 9 10 11	Wants good job recognized by others
Slow doing things	1 2 3 4 5 6 7 8 9 10 11	Fast (eating, walking)
Easy-going	1 2 3 4 5 6 7 8 9 10 11	Hard driving (pushing yourself and others)
Expresses feelings	1 2 3 4 5 6 7 8 9 10 11	Hides feelings
Many outside interests	1 2 3 4 5 6 7 8 9 10 11	Few interests outside work/home
Unambitious	1 2 3 4 5 6 7 8 9 10 11	Ambitious
Casual	1 2 3 4 5 6 7 8 9 10 11	Eager to get things done

Plot total score below:

Type B		Type A
14	84	154

├────────────┼────────────┤

Source: Cooper's adaptation of the Bortner Type A Scale

Scoring

The higher the score received on this questionnaire, the more firmly an individual can be classified as Type A. For example, 154 points is the highest score and indicates the maximum Type A coronary-prone personality. It is important to understand that there are no distinct divisions between Type A and Type B. Rather, people fall somewhere on a continuum leaning more towards one type than the other. Eighty-four is an average score. Anyone with a score above that is inclined towards Type A behaviour, and below that towards Type B behaviour.

THE 'HARDY PERSONALITY'

While the Type A/Type B distinction may provide many clues as to stress-prone personality characteristics, some researchers believe the theory is not adequate to explain why some people suffer ill health as a result of high stress levels. Suzanne Kobasa, a City University of New York researcher, developed the 'Hardy Personality' theory to explain the connection between stress and health. The theory states that 'among persons facing significant stressors, those high in hardiness will be significantly less likely to fall ill, either mentally or physically, than those who lack hardiness or who display alienation, powerlessness and threat in the face of change'.[11] The key attribute – hardiness – is defined as a personality style that expresses commitment, control and challenge. 'Commitment is the ability to believe in the truth, importance and interest of who one is and what one is doing and, thereby, the tendency to involve oneself fully in the many situations of life, including work, family, interpersonal relationships and social institutions.' Control is defined as the 'tendency to believe and act as if one can influence the course of events. Persons with control seek explanations for why something is happening with emphasis on their own responsibility and not in terms of other actions or fate.' The third aspect of the hardy personality, challenge, is based on the individual's 'belief that change, rather than stability, is the normative mode of life'. In terms of the 'challenge' aspect, an individual looks for stimulation, change, and opportunities with an openness of mind and willingness to experiment.

Kobasa suggests that hardiness leads to a type of coping. 'Keeping specific stressors in perspective, hardy individuals' basic sense of purpose in life allows them to ground events in an understandable and varied life course. Knowing that one has the resources with which to respond to stressors, hardy individuals' underlying sense of control allows them to appreciate a well-exercised coping repertoire. Seeing stressors as potential opportunities for change, challenge enables hardy individuals to see even undesirable events in terms of possibility rather than threat.'

In a retrospective study of middle- and upper-level executives, Kobasa found support for the idea that executives with high stress but low illness levels show more hardiness than similar executives with high stress and high illness levels. The healthier executives have a 'stronger commitment to self, an attitude of vigorousness toward the environment, [and] a sense of meaningfulness' than those executives suffering ill health.[12] The hardiness theory emphasizes once again the importance of the individual response to stress factors in the environment.

LOCUS OF CONTROL

One personality characteristic which may determine whether people react more or less adversely to a stressful situation is described as the 'locus of control'. The concept, first developed in the mid 1960s by J. B. Rotter, looks at the extent to which individuals feel they have control over situations.[13] Someone with an *internal* locus of control believes he or she has control over what happens, and that his or her decisions and actions influence personal outcomes. In contrast, someone with an *external* locus of control believes he or she has little influence upon situations and that outcomes are for the most part determined by fate or chance. 'Internals' are more confident that they can affect a change in the world around them, while 'Externals' believe they have little or no power to produce change. Like Type A/Type B comparisons, locus of control is not an either/or measurement, but rather a continuum between two contrasting personality types.

The locus of control theory has received a great deal of attention in recent years. Within the education field, 'internals' are frequently associated with academic success and greater motivation to achieve.[14] Studies of psychological adjustment and coping abilities have shown internals to be less anxious and better able to deal with frustration. The 'external', in contrast, appears 'less psychologically healthy'.[15] In addition, a number of studies have suggested that a person's perceived control over a situation is an advantage in managing environmental stress agents.[16] Furthermore, an internal locus of control has been found to be a major characteristic of the

Locus of Control Questionnaire

Circle the number that best reflects your attitudes:

	Strongly disagree	Disagree	Uncertain	Agree	Strongly agree
Our society is run by a few people with enormous power and there is not much the ordinary person can do about it.	1	2	3	4	5
One's success is determined by 'being in the right place at the right time'.	1	2	3	4	5
There will always be industrial relations disputes no matter how hard people try to prevent them or the extent to which they try to take an active role in union activities.	1	2	3	4	5
Politicians are inherently self-interested and inflexible. It is impossible to change the course of politics.	1	2	3	4	5
What happens in life is pre-destined.	1	2	3	4	5
People are inherently lazy, so there is no point in spending too much time in changing them.	1	2	3	4	5
I do not see a direct connection between the way and how hard I work and the assessments of my performance that others arrive at.	1	2	3	4	5
Leadership qualities are primarily inherited.	1	2	3	4	5
I am fairly certain that luck and chance play a crucial role in life.	1	2	3	4	5
Even though some people try to control events by taking part in political and social affairs, in reality most of us are subject to forces we can neither comprehend nor control.	1	2	3	4	5

Plot total score below:

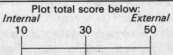

Internal		*External*
10	30	50

'hardy personality' types discussed earlier, who were able to maintain good health despite high stress levels.

It must be noted, however, that although internals' perception of control may help reduce stress in most situations, they may have even higher stress levels than externals, when presented with a situation over which they actually have no control. Therefore, the relationship between locus of control and stress responses can greatly depend upon the type of stress encountered.

The questionnaire on p. 55, based upon a scale designed by Rotter, but simplified for the purposes of this book, may be used to indicate an individual's locus of control.

Scoring

After you have filled in the questionnaire, add up all your scores. If you score a total of less than 30 points, you lean towards being an internal, while a score above 30 would indicate an external orientation. Obviously, your specific orientation will depend on the *degree* of your score, with 10 points at the internal and 50 at the external end-points respectively.

COPING STRATEGIES

The way an individual copes with a stress agent, once he or she has perceived it as such, becomes an integral part of his or her 'vulnerability profile'. Inappropriate coping strategies may actually add to the stress experienced; the desire to deal with a threat inappropriately, for instance, might also prove stressful and set off a spiral of effects. It is helpful to recognize that coping is not only a reaction to stress; coping can be preventive by anticipating a stressful situation.

To better comprehend what an individual can do to meet the pressures he or she encounters, it is important to understand the *coping process* itself. At first, the individual *identifies* a set of pressures as stressful; he (or she) feels anxious, unable to cope and exhibits his own characteristic pattern of physical and mental symptoms of stress and defensive behaviour. This reaction is described by Richard Lazarus [17] as a period of 'shock', during which the individual builds up strength to face the future. The behaviour which then follows this period of 'protective withdrawal' can be described as either adaptive or maladaptive. Adaptive behaviour deals directly with the stressful situation by seeking and implementing solutions. It not only deals with the immediate problem, but can give the individual a well-earned sense of achievement and help prepare him or her to deal with similar situations in the future. For this reason, adaptive behaviour is seen as being *developmental* in nature. On the other hand, maladaptive behaviour does not deal directly with the problem faced. Maladaptive behaviour is defensive in nature – it aims at removing the stressful situation, but usually only achieves this result temporarily. It often does not remove the anxiety felt by the individual; neither does it prepare him or her to deal with future problems. Maladaptive coping techniques can range from simple procrastination or denial that a problem exists, to more blatantly poor coping efforts such as overdrinking.

As Figure 1 shows, an individual who is dealing actively with his environment, both making and receiving demands, can reach a point where the particular combination of demands is perceived as stressful: i.e., the individual feels unable to cope. Following the period of defensive behaviour, this person adopts a type of behaviour, either adaptive or maladaptive. As the diagram shows, up to a certain point (B), maladaptive behaviour can be abandoned for adaptive behaviour, leading to a positive result. After point B, negative consequences such as psychological distress, work or family disruptions cannot be compensated for by successful coping.[18]

Further research indicates that people use different methods of coping for different stress agents, and the selection of inappropriate strategies can become a critical factor within each situation. Some research has found that the immune system may be adversely affected by maladaptive coping strategies. In a study of more than 2,100 women attending breast screening clinics, it was found that women who keep 'emotional material' buried (particularly during periods involving stressful events such as the loss of a loved one) are significantly more at risk from breast cancer than those who are able to express their feelings, to seek help and to acknowledge the underlying stress-related event.[19] The following questionnaire is similar to that used in the breast cancer study and may give an indication of how well you are able to cope with a

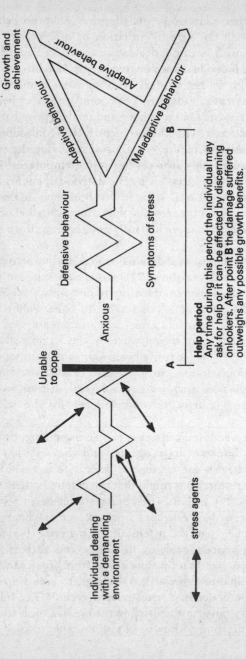

Figure 1. The Coping Process
Source: C. L. Cooper and J. Marshall, 'The Management of Stress', *Personnel Review*, Autumn 1975.

Coping With Life Stress

The purpose of this questionnaire is to find out how people deal with situations which trouble them.

Take a few moments and think about an event or situation which has been most stressful to you. By 'stressful' we mean a serious situation which was difficult, troubling or upsetting to you. It might have been something to do with your family, your friends, your spouse or children.

Thinking about the situation, to what extent do you do the following:

Temporary Adaptation

	Never	Rarely	Periodically	Regularly	Very often
Get on with work, keep busy	1	2	3	4	5
Throw yourself into work	1	2	3	4	5
Do some housework	1	2	3	4	5
Try to do something where you don't use your mind	1	2	3	4	5
Cry on your own	1	2	3	4	5
Bottle it up for a time, then break down	1	2	3	4	5
Explosive, mostly temper, not tears	1	2	3	4	5
Treat yourself to something, e.g. clothes, meals out	1	2	3	4	5

Adaptive Behaviour

	Never	Rarely	Periodically	Regularly	Very often
Sit and think	1	2	3	4	5
Ability to cry with friends	1	2	3	4	5
Get angry with people or things which cause the problem	1	2	3	4	5
Let feelings out, talk to close friends	1	2	3	4	5
Talk things over with lots of friends	1	2	3	4	5
Go over the problem again and again in your mind to try to understand it	1	2	3	4	5
Feel you learn something from every distress	1	2	3	4	5

	Never	Rarely	Periodically	Regularly	Very often
Talk to someone who could do something about the problem	1	2	3	4	5
Try to get sympathy and understanding from someone	1	2	3	4	5

Maladaptive Behaviour

	Never	Rarely	Periodically	Regularly	Very often
Try not to think about it	5	4	3	2	1
Go quiet	5	4	3	2	1
Go on as if nothing happened	5	4	3	2	1
Keep feelings to yourself	5	4	3	2	1
Avoid being with people	5	4	3	2	1
Show a 'brave face'	5	4	3	2	1
Worry constantly	5	4	3	2	1
Lose sleep	5	4	3	2	1
Don't eat	5	4	3	2	1
Control tears (hide feelings)	5	4	3	2	1
Eat more	5	4	3	2	1
Wish that you could change what happened	5	4	3	2	1
Have fantasies or wishes about how things might have turned out	5	4	3	2	1

Plot total score below:

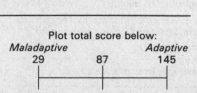

Maladaptive		Adaptive
29	87	145

Coping With Work Stress

When you have a work-related problem or stress to what extent do you do the following:

Adaptive Behaviour	Never	Rarely	Periodically	Regularly	Very often
Seek support and advice from supervisors	1	2	3	4	5
Try to deal with the situation objectively in an unemotional way	1	2	3	4	5
Try to recognize your own limitations	1	2	3	4	5
Talk to understanding colleagues	1	2	3	4	5
Set priorities and deal with problems accordingly	1	2	3	4	5
Accept the situation and learn to live with it	1	2	3	4	5
Seek as much social support as possible	1	2	3	4	5

Maladaptive Behaviour					
'Staying busy'	5	4	3	2	1
'Bottling things up'	5	4	3	2	1
Using distractions (to take your mind off things)	5	4	3	2	1
Smoking more	5	4	3	2	1
Delegate the problem	5	4	3	2	1
Drink alcohol rather more than usual	5	4	3	2	1
Try to avoid the situation	5	4	3	2	1

Plot total score below:

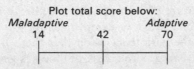

Maladaptive   *Adaptive*
14   42   70

stressful event or situation. This is followed by a second questionnaire for those interested in work-related issues.

Both of the following questionnaires show that the more often you use maladaptive coping strategies in contrast to adaptive ones, the more likely the health outcomes and other stress manifestations will be negative. The longer you use these maladaptive behaviours, the worse the behavioural and health prognosis and the more distant the long-term solution to the underlying cause of stress.

LIFE EVENTS

One's vulnerability to stress can be influenced by events in life which cause undue emotional strain. Simply encountering a significant degree of change, even positive change, in a relatively short period of time is believed to raise stress levels. It is important to realize that the amount of change that is taking place in your life may be causing you irreparable harm. These can stem from factors beyond your control, such as the death of a close relative, and to some which you are party to (either wittingly or involuntarily), such as divorce, pregnancy, and so on.

A considerable body of research in the last fifteen years suggests that life changes are a determining factor in stress-related illnesses. American researchers at Washington University in St Louis conducted a survey from which they calculated the relative amounts of 'social adjustment' required after certain life events.[20] They then applied these weightings (that is, evaluations of the degree of seriousness of each life event on a 100-point scale) to the events in the lives of sample populations and arrived at 'life change scores' for a given period. In their studies, they found high life change scores to be related to the onset of illness within the following two-year period.

Other studies also purport to show that the greater the life change experienced, the more serious the disease which develops, and that an increase in life events was associated with worsening symptoms, a decrease with improvement.[22] These researchers contend that the nature of the change – whether it is favourable or unfavourable, competitive or complementary – is immaterial.

Although the basic conclusion that there is a link between changes in life events and the onset of illness is generally accepted, questionnaires which attempt to measure the effects of these changes have some flaws. For example, most questionnaires list a number of events which may be symptoms or consequences of illness rather than other critical life events (for example, a change in the number of marital arguments, dismissal from work, sexual difficulties, etc.) Secondly, the illness itself may impede or prevent someone from accurately recalling past events. But by far the most important drawback of the questionnaires lies in the fact that individual perceptions of the events are not taken into account. Each life event listed in a scale may have a different meaning for each person questioned, but they are rigidly weighted. In the large-scale study undertaken by Cary and Rachel Cooper on the link between psychological and social stress and breast cancer, they discovered early on that the scale of stress attributed to particular life events frequently failed to correspond with individual perceptions of the severity of such events. In the design of their prospective study, they incorporated, therefore, a 10-point rating scale for each life event, based on its degree of upset or stressfulness to the individual. They found that there were substantial differences between the cancer patients' perceptions of these events and the perceptions of women who were well. (Note that these perceptions were recorded on the first visit to the clinic and well in advance of the diagnosis of cancer.) If a standard 'life events' scale had been used, the healthy women and those with cancer would have been seen to have sustained roughly the same impact from life events, even though the cancer patients may have perceived the events as roughly twice as stressful as the other women. Indeed, they found that of the 42 items in the Cooper, Cooper and Cheang Life Events Scale, cancer patients perceived themselves to be significantly more stressed than the well-women control group on 29 items.

It should be remembered, also, that items on any life events scale should relate specifically to the people being questioned. For example, it has been found that items described as significantly stressful by American women differed from those described by English women. Here again, a scale which allows each person to rate the *degree* of stress felt by a particular event takes individual perceptions into account.

The following life stress inventory can help measure life change and susceptibility to stress-related illness. Although the scale can give some indication of the probability of health breakdown based on the number of simultaneously occurring stressful events, it does not take into account a number of important factors. The extent to which these events lead to ill health will depend to a large degree on a person's capacity to cope with stress, on the personal support the individual has and how important each life event is perceived to be. It can, however, give one an idea of how stress factors, which arise with changes in life, are being experienced by the individual, and act as a warning sign for a potentially stressful situation.

Life Events

Place a cross (X) in the 'Yes' column for each event which has taken place in the last two years. Then circle a number on the scale which best describes how upsetting the event crossed was to you, e.g. 10 for death of husband.

Event	Yes	Scale
Bought house		1 2 3 4 5 6 7 8 9 10
Sold house		1 2 3 4 5 6 7 8 9 10
Moved house		1 2 3 4 5 6 7 8 9 10
Major house renovation		1 2 3 4 5 6 7 8 9 10
Separation from loved one		1 2 3 4 5 6 7 8 9 10
End of relationship		1 2 3 4 5 6 7 8 9 10
Got engaged		1 2 3 4 5 6 7 8 9 10
Got married		1 2 3 4 5 6 7 8 9 10
Marital problem		1 2 3 4 5 6 7 8 9 10
Awaiting divorce		1 2 3 4 5 6 7 8 9 10
Divorce		1 2 3 4 5 6 7 8 9 10
Child started school/nursery		1 2 3 4 5 6 7 8 9 10
Increased nursing responsibilities for elderly or sick person		1 2 3 4 5 6 7 8 9 10

Event	Yes	Scale
Problems with relatives		1 2 3 4 5 6 7 8 9 10
Problems with friends/ neighbours		1 2 3 4 5 6 7 8 9 10
Pet-related problems		1 2 3 4 5 6 7 8 9 10
Work-related problems		1 2 3 4 5 6 7 8 9 10
Change in nature of work		1 2 3 4 5 6 7 8 9 10
Threat of redundancy		1 2 3 4 5 6 7 8 9 10
Changed job		1 2 3 4 5 6 7 8 9 10
Made redundant		1 2 3 4 5 6 7 8 9 10
Unemployed		1 2 3 4 5 6 7 8 9 10
Retired		1 2 3 4 5 6 7 8 9 10
Increased or new bank loan/mortgage		1 2 3 4 5 6 7 8 9 10
Financial difficulty		1 2 3 4 5 6 7 8 9 10
Insurance problem		1 2 3 4 5 6 7 8 9 10
Legal problem		1 2 3 4 5 6 7 8 9 10
Emotional or physical illness of close family or relative		1 2 3 4 5 6 7 8 9 10
Serious illness of close family or relative requiring hospitalization		1 2 3 4 5 6 7 8 9 10
Surgical operation experienced by family member or relative		1 2 3 4 5 6 7 8 9 10
Death of husband		1 2 3 4 5 6 7 8 9 10
Death of family member or relative		1 2 3 4 5 6 7 8 9 10
Death of close friend		1 2 3 4 5 6 7 8 9 10

Event	Yes	Scale
Emotional or physical illness of yourself		1 2 3 4 5 6 7 8 9 10
Serious illness requiring your own hospitalization		1 2 3 4 5 6 7 8 9 10
Surgical operation on yourself		1 2 3 4 5 6 7 8 9 10
Pregnancy		1 2 3 4 5 6 7 8 9 10
Birth of baby		1 2 3 4 5 6 7 8 9 10
Birth of grandchild		1 2 3 4 5 6 7 8 9 10
Family member left home		1 2 3 4 5 6 7 8 9 10
Difficult relationship with children		1 2 3 4 5 6 7 8 9 10
Difficult relationship with parents		1 2 3 4 5 6 7 8 9 10

Plot total score below:

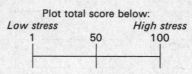

Many researchers believe that our differences according to age, sex and ethnic background may make some individuals more vulnerable to the negative effects of stress. Some of the theories are described below.

AGE

We have already discussed how an individual's perception of a threat can play a major part in setting up a stressful scenario. The degree to which an event is perceived as a threat can often depend upon the age of the person involved. For example, a young, confident manager may see the merger of his or her firm with a large conglomerate as offering exciting opportunities, while an older person may see it as a potential threat to his or her job and therefore a far greater stress factor. Also, stress-related symptoms or illnesses may often be determined by the biological age of the person involved. As James and Jonathan Quick suggest, a younger man 'may respond with an imperceptible rise in pulse and blood pressure, while an older executive with many years of high cholesterol and cigarette smoking behind him may experience severe chest pain or even a heart attack'.[23]

It is widely believed that 'mid-life crisis' increases one's sensitivity to life in general and to stress in particular. Most research in this area has been conducted on men; the mid-life crisis is seen to affect them regardless of occupation. As one researcher suggests, it seems to be 'a period of particular vulnerability, a time of low resistance when a combination of other forces, internal and external, can torment a person in a way that would not have bothered that individual when younger'.[24] Alan McLean describes graphically a man in mid-life crisis:

At forty-one Amos McPherson had become his own person but he was ripe for mid-life transition. Indeed, as he thought to himself, everything was going too well! He had, for two years, had staff responsibility for a major company function in the suburban headquarters of a large manufacturer. He had autonomy, the respect of his colleagues and superiors, and a substantial salary and stock-option plan. He and his family felt that their life was stable, secure. His sons, aged fifteen and thirteen, were doing well in school. His wife enjoyed a comfortable routine with part-time work as an editor and an active social and cultural life.

Yet the 'impossible' happened. McPherson's company merged with one of equal size. Duplicate staff functions were eliminated in the successor organization and McPherson was out – overnight, unexpectedly.

After a period of overtly expressed anger, McPherson became depressed. While he was not seriously disabled, he did have symptoms of irritability, frustration, insomnia, and, increasingly, bowel and stomach disorders. His new job required a long commute and left much less time for his family and avocational interests and it stimulated a searching evaluation of his occupational goals. This reassessment, however, led only to increasing frustration. He blamed himself for not seeing the potential threat and not getting his 'ducks lined up' outside in order to step into a higher rather than lower job level with another organization. He felt locked into his present job; that he was not in a position to look elsewhere 'because I couldn't really sell myself now'.

These same seeds of self-doubt permeated all aspects of his life. He questioned the future viability of his marriage, which did indeed begin to founder leading to eventual separation and divorce.

Women also can find the middle years vulnerable as they often have to deal with changing roles after children are grown. They often succeed in finding new things to occupy their time, such as demanding jobs, which shift their relationships. While such changes can provide exciting results for many, other women may experience relationship problems and even divorce, leaving them particularly vulnerable at times.

Old age and retirement can be a time of increased stress vulnerability for those who have not adapted well to life change and developed new interests. Also, the loss of friends and loved ones during this time can, of course, be especially difficult if other support is not present.

SEX

Until recently, men have been more at risk from stress-related illnesses than women. A man's life expectancy is eight years less than a woman's. This may be partly biological and partly due to the male lifestyle, which often includes more Type A behaviour, and higher consumption of cigarettes and alcohol. But, as discussed in Chapter 2, women are developing many of the same patterns of dealing with stress factors in their lives. The increased dependence of women on a range of coping mechanisms may reflect the growing demands and potential conflicts of work and home life. In addition, studies by Cary Cooper and Marilyn Davidson[25] have shown there are a number of sources of stress in society that adversely affect women more than men, such as expectations of child-rearing, male attitudes towards working women, lack of resource support for working mothers, etc.

ETHNICITY AND CULTURAL BACKGROUND

Minority groups in any society have the additional problems of stress resulting from racial prejudice, which may appear both in social and work settings. Changing roles and expectations of minorities can also leave individuals with reduced social structure and support. For example, when someone from a minority group moves into a supervisory or management job held previously only by whites, no successful role models or mentors will be available to offer support. Members of cultural subgroups can encounter stressors in situations where they feel in the minority or where their belief systems clash with predominant attitudes and values.

OCCUPATION

Although we will examine work stress in detail in the next chapter, it is important to note that the simple choice of occupation may make daily life intrinsically more stressful, and as a result increase vulnerability to stress and its health consequences. An independent panel of stress research experts was asked to rate the degree of job stress in nearly one hundred occupations. It was found that journalists, pilots, miners, police officers and many others were in high-stress occupations, while museum keepers, physicists, and biologists were in relatively low-stress jobs. A further look at the relationship between various occupations and stress will be taken in Chapter 4.

PREFERRED PATTERNS OF PSYCHOPHYSIOLOGICAL RESPONSES

All individuals have a particular way of responding to high levels of environmental stimulation or stress. This predisposition may be genetic or biological in nature or may result from learned family patterns. One person may respond to stress agents with a churning stomach, while another's cardiovascular system may be disturbed. As medical researcher, Harold Wolff, wrote in the 1950s: 'A given protective pattern may remain inconspicuous during long periods of relative security, and then with stress, becomes evident as a disorder involving the gut, the heart and vascular system, the vaso-respiratory system, the skin or general metabolism.'[26]

SOCIAL SUPPORT

Each individual meets the world daily with a complex set of physical and emotional characteristics, coping styles, values and particular history. This 'individual vulnerability' forms the first part of the *stress equation*, as he or she prepares to meet his or her environment, its satisfactions and pressures. Despite the importance of this individual make-up, studies today show that a positive and nurturing support group, such as family, friends and co-workers, can offset many of the effects of stress and coronary heart disease.

An important study in 1975 looked at the differences between Japanese and American cultures in terms of social support and stress.[27] At the time of this study, it had already been shown that the high-fat diet of Americans contributed substantially to their incidence of coronary heart disease, while the much lower intake of fats in the diets of Japanese seemed to reduce their risk substantially. The 1975 study attempted to see if there were other social factors involved in the much lower Japanese mortality rates due to heart disease. The study looked at 11,991 men of Japanese ancestry (2,141 living in Japan, 8,006 in Hawaii, and 1,844 in California). The study was designed to eliminate age factors and to control for high-fat diets. It was found that the prevalence of coronary heart disease increased from Japan to Hawaii, and again from Hawaii to California, where it was approximately double the rate in Japan. The known risk factors of hypertension, serum cholesterol levels and smoking were roughly the same in all three regions, so could not be used to explain the rising prevalence of coronary heart disease as one approached the United States. The investigators concluded that the acculturation of the Japanese, that is, the extent to which they have abandoned their traditional way of life and moved towards the American model of a mobile nuclear family, may explain the differences. The researchers suggested that the more hectic, demanding pace of the United States, together with the lack of social supports such as the extended family and a stable community of friends, are to blame.

In another study, it was seen that among a group of un-employed workers, individuals who lacked social support from family, friends and the community had significantly more symptoms of emotional and physical ill health than did those with support. They had a notably higher serum cholesterol count (a coronary heart disease risk factor), were depressed, reported more illnesses and perceived economic deprivation.[28]

It is clear that a husband or wife and the immediate family can be a major source of support. They provide the problem-solving, listening and acceptance that can relieve stress even though they may not be able to solve the related problems. One study of 190 engineers or accountants and their wives showed that the more compatible the husbands and wives were, the higher the likelihood that the men could cope better with stress-related problems at work and home.[29] Studies of Norwegian prisoners of war in Nazi concentration camps showed that close social support was essential to their survival. Individuals who had been able to retain close ties with family, friends and religious or political groups survived more often and were best able to adjust to normal life when freed.[30]

THE FAMILY AS SUPPORT SYSTEM

A useful approach to understanding how the family acts as a support system was outlined by G. Caplan in 1967.[31] Caplan suggested that the family serves a number of different roles for the individual: a collector and disseminator of information about the world; a feedback/guidance system; a source of ideology; a guide and mediator in problem-solving; a source of practical service and concrete aid; a haven for rest and recuperation; a reference and control group.

The family provides its members with a history of how to cope; of how members lived, worked and dealt with the problems of human existence. This was done much better by the close extended family of years past; each family member had a wider pool of experience available to help advise about the world.

The family provides feedback on members' behaviour, experiences and feelings. As Caplan explains, during a typical family meal, for example, family members interpret the day's events for one another, putting experiences in the context of family or societal values. The family acts as a mirror of our own values and behaviours and is a tremendous source of support and 'reality testing'.

In addition, the family is a source of ideology, providing the belief systems and norms of behaviour that determine an individual's understanding of the nature of the world. This structure can assist with crucial personal decisions facing each of us. As problem-solvers, family members can provide guidance, mediation, opinions and often, practical assistance such as babysitting, repair work or financial aid. Finally, one of the most important roles of the family is as a haven for rest and recuperation. The family can provide a sanctuary for failures and disappointments, a place where the family member is accepted as himself. Although few families perfectly provide all of the qualities described above, they often act as a powerful force for support and change. In this way the family can be a strong buffer between an individual and potential outside stress agents. Conversely, if the family poorly supports its members or, indeed, acts as a source of stress itself, the individual could be considered more susceptible to stress.

SOCIAL SUPPORT AT WORK

Home life is not the only form of social support. For many people, their co-workers act as a sort of substitute family group. A person's boss or supervisor can provide the critical feedback and support necessary to enhance mental well-being, while co-workers may provide the friendship and camaraderie helpful in stressful situations. An active level of participation at work appears to provide the social support that inoculates people against stress. As early as the 1940s, researchers explored the effects of involvement at work, discovering that the greater the participation, the higher the productivity, the greater the job satisfaction, the lower the staff turnover, and the better the relationships between boss and subordinates.[32] Figure 2 illustrates the effect of 'participation' as a support system in the workplace.

A study of NASA personnel found that people who reported greater opportunities for participation in decision-making reported significantly greater job satisfaction, lower job-related feelings of threat, and higher feelings of self-esteem.[33] Another study of more than 1,400 US workers found that non-participation and the absence of support systems at work were the most consistent and significant predictors or indicators of strain and job-related stress. They found that non-participation was significantly related to the following health risk factors: low self-esteem, low life and job satisfaction,

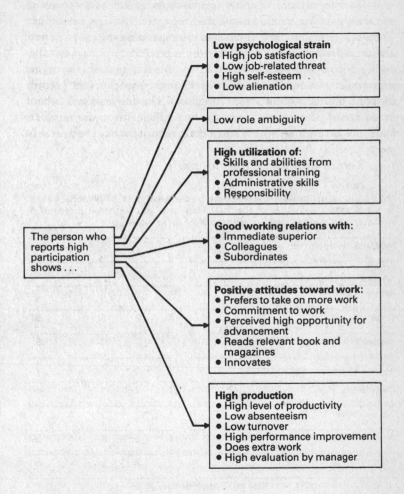

**Figure 2. The Effect of Involvement
in the Workplace**
Source: J. R. P. French and R. D. Caplan, 'Organizational Stress and
Individual Strain', in *The Failure of Success*, ed. A. J. Marrow
(New York: A M A C O M, 1973), p. 52

escapist drinking, low motivation to work, and increased absenteeism and intentions to leave work.[34]

The importance of the informal work group as a source of social support was validated in a study of 3,725 US Navy personnel. The study, which looked at enlisted men spanning the range of pay grades, determined that support from a boss and co-workers was both positive and accumulative in its impact, that is, the more support one obtained from one's leader and co-workers the greater the reduction in manifestations of stress.[35] The desire to seek others in situations of danger or stress is not difficult to understand. In many instances, man appears to obtain security from the nearness

Social Support Questionnaire

Personal Problems
Think of a situation which has caused you a great deal of personal stress. To what extent did each of the following help you with the problem? 1 indicates little support and 5 a great deal of social support.

Husband/wife, partner	1	2	3	4	5
Mother	1	2	3	4	5
Father	1	2	3	4	5
Sister	1	2	3	4	5
Brother	1	2	3	4	5
Other relative	1	2	3	4	5
Close friend	1	2	3	4	5
Casual friend	1	2	3	4	5
Work colleague	1	2	3	4	5
Doctor/clergyman/counsellor	1	2	3	4	5

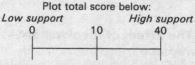

Plot total score below:
Low support   *High support*
0   10   40

Note: a positive score is 10, when one person is assigned 3 or more on the scale.

Work Problems

Think of a situation at work which has caused you a great deal of stress. To what extent did each of the following help you with the problem?

Husband/wife, partner	1	2	3	4	5
Mother	1	2	3	4	5
Father	1	2	3	4	5
Sister	1	2	3	4	5
Brother	1	2	3	4	5
Other relative	1	2	3	4	5
Close friend	1	2	3	4	5
Casual friend	1	2	3	4	5
Boss	1	2	3	4	5
Colleague	1	2	3	4	5
Subordinate	1	2	3	4	5
Doctor/clergyman/counsellor	1	2	3	4	5

Plot total score below:

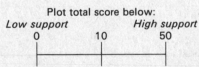

Low support   *High support*

0   10   50

Note: a positive score is 10, when one person is assigned 3 or more on the scale.

of others; the larger the pack, the fewer the animals that fall prey to predators.[36] The complicated set of relationships at work, and their potential for conflict and ambiguity, leads individuals to seek support from their peers in informal support systems.

It is important to note that the best social support is that which helps the individual identify a problem and sort it out. Poor social support involves colluding with someone to maintain an inaccurate view of the problem. For example, family support may help a member through a crisis by shielding that individual from bad news; in this case the family may act as a buffer to protect the person rather than force him or her to confront the problem at a difficult time. Work support can sometimes help push a person to deal with a problem directly.

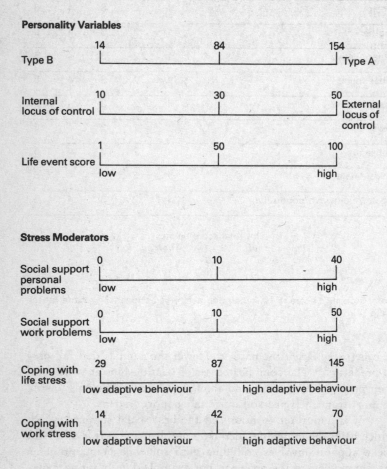

Personality Variables

Type B — 14 — 84 — 154 Type A

Internal locus of control — 10 — 30 — 50 External locus of control

Life event score — 1 low — 50 — 100 high

Stress Moderators

Social support personal problems — 0 low — 10 — 40 high

Social support work problems — 0 low — 10 — 50 high

Coping with life stress — 29 low adaptive behaviour — 87 — 145 high adaptive behaviour

Coping with work stress — 14 low adaptive behaviour — 42 — 70 high adaptive behaviour

Figure 3. Vulnerability Profile

OVERALL VULNERABILITY PROFILE

As we have described in this chapter, the individual's vulnerability to stress is composed of a number of complex factors – personality, coping strategies, personal history and social support. The self-assessment questionnaires throughout this chapter may give you an indication of your own vulnerability in these areas. By plotting the scores on to the Vulnerability Profile (Figure 3), you will be able to get a rough idea of your overall vulnerability. Figure 4 illustrates possible profiles: a *high vulnerability* may mean that you have vulnerable personality characteristics and no coping mechanisms (such as stress moderators), whereas a *low vulnerability* profile suggests strong personality characteristics, and good stress moderators. Someone with strong personality variables but poor stress moderators, must be concerned if he or she is ever faced with a stressful event or situation. On the other hand, the person who already has weak personality characteristics (suggesting, perhaps, some stressful life events or an extreme Type A personality), may be coping well, if his or her profile indicates good stress moderators. Chapters 4 and 5 will discuss the environmental factors which help complete your 'stress equation'.

78 · *Living with Stress*

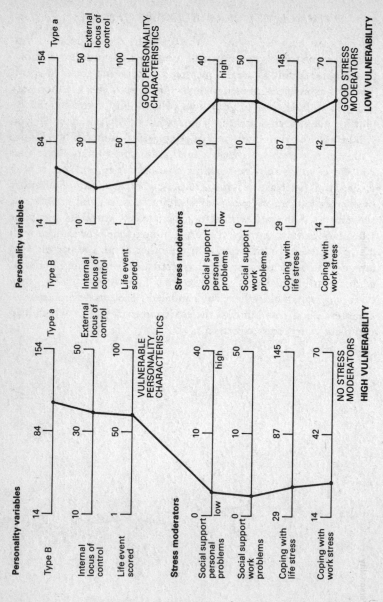

Figure 4. Vulnerability Profiles

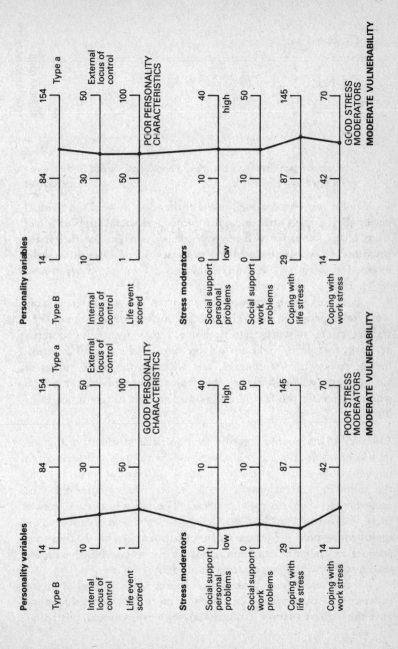

Chapter Four

STRESS AND WORK

'The reason why worry kills more people than work is that more
people worry than work'   Robert Frost

In the last chapter, we looked at the ways in which individual
personality, coping strategies, life events and social support affect
stress levels. Now we will move to the second part of the 'stress
equation' – the environment. As discussed in Chapter 1, it is the
interaction between the individual and his or her environment
which leads to the stress response.

Because a high proportion of women, as well as men, now
work, most people in our industrialized society spend more of their
waking hours at work than at home. Stress agents encountered
at work, therefore, make up a large part of the overall environmental stress. In this chapter, we will examine work stress; in
Chapter 5 we will look at the other major aspects of environmental
stress – stress in the family and stress faced at different stages of
life.

Although many people describe their work as stressful, it appears
that some occupations carry more stress than others. Little research
has been done to compare stress levels of different occupations, but
the following 'stress league' table ranks over a hundred jobs
according to their degrees of stress.[1] The table is drawn from a
survey performed by leading stress researchers and based upon
their professional judgements of occupational stress. It takes into
account available health trend evidence and is combined with research from occupational stress literature.

It is interesting to look at the average stress ratings of broad
occupational categories. For instance, the uniformed professions
have the highest average ratings (6.4), with policemen in particular

Table 1. The Cooper Occupational Stress Ratings†
In order of the most stressful groups of jobs:
*** extremely stressful job
** very stressful job
* above average stressful job

1. Uniformed professions

Armed forces	4.7
Civil aviation (pilot)	7.5***
Merchant navy	4.8
Fire brigade	6.3**
Police force	7.7***
Prison service	7.5***
Ambulance service	6.3**
Average	6.4

2. Arts and communications

Art and design	4.2
Broadcasting	6.8**
Journalism	7.5***
Museum personnel	2.8
Photographer	4.6
Publishing	5.0*
Musician	6.3**
Acting	7.2***
Film production	6.5**
Professional sport	5.8*
Librarian	2.0
Average	5.3

3. Commerce/management

Advertising	7.3***
Management	5.8*
Marketing/export	5.8*
Market research	4.3
Personnel	6.0**
Public relations	5.8*
Purchasing and supply	4.5
Sales and retailing	5.7*
Secretary	4.7*
Company secretary	5.3*
Work study/O and M	3.6
Average	5.3

4. Industrial production

Ceramic technology	4.0
Food technology	4.0
Printing	5.6*
Plastics and rubber	4.5
Textiles/clothing technology	4.5
Timber/furniture technology	4.3

Leather/footwear technology	3.8
Mining	8.3***
Construction/building	7.5***
Brewing	4.0
Average	5.1

5. Caring professions

Nursery nursing	3.3
Social work	6.0**
Teaching	6.2**
Youth and community work	4.2
Church	3.5
Psychologist	5.2*
Average	4.7

6. Health

Chiropody	4.0
Dentistry	7.3***
Dietetics	3.4
Environmental health	4.6
Doctor	6.8**
Nursing/midwifery	6.5**
Occupational therapy	3.7
Optician	4.0
Osteopath	4.3

Pharmacist	4.5
Vet	4.5
Physiotherapy	4.2
Radiographer	4.0
Remedial gymnast	3.5
Speech therapy	4.0
Average	4.6

7. Personal service industries

Catering/hotel business, etc.	5.3*
Travel industry	4.8
Hairdressing	4.3
Beauty therapy	3.5
Average	4.5

8. Public service industries

Post and telecommunications	4.0
Gas	4.0
Electricity	4.6
Water	4.0
Public transport	5.4*
Average	4.5

9. Professional services

Architect	4.0

Barrister	5.7*
Solicitor	4.3
Surveyor	4.3
Estate agent	4.3
Average	4.4

10. Public administration

Civil service	4.4
Diplomatic service	4.8
Local government	4.3
Town and country planning	4.0
Sports/recreation admin.	3.5
Average	4.2

11. Financial areas

Accountancy	4.3
Banking	3.7
Building societies	3.3
Insurance	3.8
Actuary	3.3
Stockbroker	5.5*
Average	4.0

12. Environment

Farming	4.8
Forestry	4.8
Horticulture	3.8
Nature conservancy	3.2
Average	3.9

13. Technical specialities

Biologist	3.0
Chemist	3.7
Computer programmer	3.8
Engineer	4.3
Geologist	3.7
Laboratory technician	3.8
Metallurgist	3.8
Operational researcher	3.8
Packaging	3.8
Patent work	4.2
Physicist	3.4
Biochemist	3.6
Statistician	4.0
Linguist	3.6
Astronomer	3.4
Average	3.7

† Six experienced stress researchers independently evaluated each job on a 10-point scale, from least stressful (1) to most stressful (10). Each score represents the mean average of these ratings.

(Professor Cooper was originally commissioned to carry out these ratings by the *Sunday Times*, and he would like to thank them for their support and encouragement.)

coming out on top (7.7). Arts/communication and commerce/ management tie for second place with an average of 5.3, and among them actors, journalists and advertisers are most 'at risk'. Among the other professional groupings averaging 4.7 or above are health care professionals such as dentists, nurses and doctors. (These and other professionals will be discussed in more detail in this chapter.)

Evidence that stress-related illnesses are not the exclusive problem of either high- or low-status workers was the result of a study conducted by the US National Institute of Occupational Safety and Health.[2] In the investigation, the health records of 22,000 Tennessee workers admitted to mental hospitals due to stress-related illnesses were examined. It was found that managers, foremen, office workers as well as waitresses had a high incidence of stress-related illness. As one researcher summarized the report, 'occupational status level has no relationship to the incidence of stress-related disease. Both white- and blue-collar employees showed high and low incidence of stress-related disease. Managers, foremen, and shopfloor employees all showed high and low incidence; skilled and unskilled workers also showed both high and low incidence.'[3]

Regardless of how one job may compare to another in terms of stress, it is helpful to recognize that every job has potential stress agents. Researchers have identified five major categories of work stress.[4] Common to all jobs, these factors vary in the degree to which they are found to be casually linked to stress in each job. The five categories are:

1 Factors intrinsic to the job
2 Role in the organization
3 Relationships at work
4 Career development
5 Organizational structure and climate

As we examine each of these categories, you may want to consider whether the stress agents included in each category are present in your personal work situation.

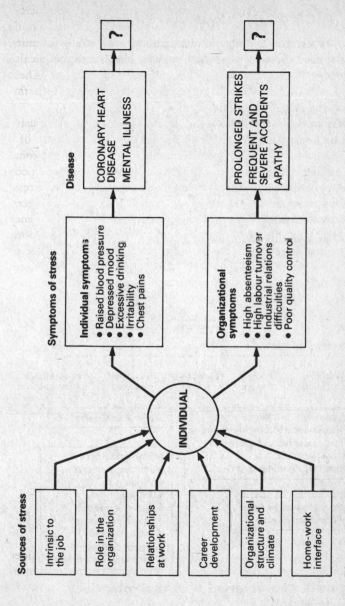

Figure 1. Dynamics of Work Stress

FACTORS INTRINSIC TO THE JOB

As a starting point to understanding work stress, researchers have studied those factors which may be intrinsic to the job itself, such as:

1 Poor working conditions
2 Shift work
3 Long hours
4 Travel
5 Risk and danger
6 New technology
7 Work overload
8 Work underload

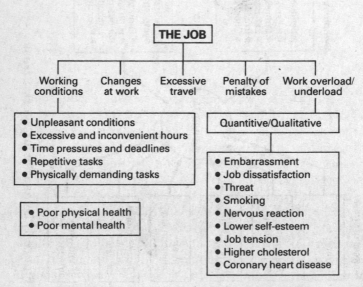

Figure 2. Characteristics of the Potentially Stressful Job

Working Conditions

Our physical surroundings – noise, lighting, smells and all the stimuli which bombard our senses – can affect our moods and overall mental state, whether or not we find them consciously objectionable. Considerable research has linked working conditions to mental health. One study found, for example, that 'poor mental health was directly related to unpleasant working conditions, the necessity to work fast and to expend a lot of physical effort, and to excessive and inconvenient hours'.[5] Others have found that physical health is also adversely affected by repetitive and dehumanizing work settings, such as fast-paced assembly lines. In one study of stress agents associated with casting work in a steel manufacturing plant, poor working conditions such as noise, fumes and to a lesser extent, heat, together with the social and psychological consequences of isolation and tension among workers, had significant impact.[6] One result was low job satisfaction, which was exacerbated by the nature of the task of casting liquid steel in a continuous process lasting seventy minutes. For three-quarters of this time period, the casters were unable to move away from very high noise levels (up to 110 decibels), and unpleasant air pollution caused by the activities of other workers and nearby machines. These conditions caused workers to wear ear protection such as ear muffs or cotton wool swabs, which effectively isolated them from each other.

Health workers, too, often face a variety of noxious stimuli. Hospital lighting, for example, is usually artificial, monotonous, and too bright or garish. One study of the problems experienced by nurses working in intensive care units in the US found that an oppressive visual environment became particularly stressful to nurses over a period of time.[7] This factor, combined with the incessant routine nature of many of the activities, led to feelings of being trapped, of claustrophobia and dehumanization. As the authors conclude, 'eventually the nurse begins to feel like a hamster on a tread mill'. Nurses have also identified bad smells as potential stress agents, although workers often acquire an immunity to them. Poor ventilating systems worsen the problem in many hospitals. In addition, the high noise level of a busy ward adds to the stress factors faced by health professionals. All of this, of course, is in addition to the stress encountered in dealing daily with death and pain.[8]

Each occupation has its own potential environmental sources of stress. For example, in jobs where individuals are dealing with close detail work, poor lighting can create eye strain. On the other hand, extremely bright lighting or glare presents problems for air traffic controllers. Similarly, as Ivancevich and Matteson state, 'noise, in fact, seems to operate less as a stressor in situations where it is excessive but expected, than in those where it is unexpected, or at least unpredictable. The change in noise levels more than absolute levels themselves, seems to be the irritant. This, of course, is simply another way of saying that noise, like any stressor, causes stress when it forces us to change.'[9]

Temperature, too, can be a part of environmental stress. In most working environments today, temperature is carefully controlled. However, there are some work sites where it cannot be controlled, such as a steel mill or pottery kilns. Regions which have temperature extremes offer challenges for construction workers, and outdoor workers naturally face uncontrolled temperatures. Ivancevich and Matteson state that 'excessive heat is a potential stressor likely to generate both physiological and psychological costs, particularly to those engaged in heavy physical activities. Physiologically, heat stress results in increased blood flow and heart rate, higher oxygen demands and fatigue; psychologically, it can disrupt normal effective functioning and greatly increase irritability.' They also point out that extreme cold can affect energy levels and possibly decrease motivation.

All of the above environmental factors can lead to secondary stress effects, that is, the knowledge that *what* you are working with may have long-term detrimental effects on health and well-being. For example, an asbestos worker 'may experience stress each day because of the knowledge that the asbestos he or she is exposed to may appreciably reduce the chance of living a healthy, normal life span'.[10]

The design or physical setting of the workplace can be another potential source of stress. If an office is poorly designed, with personnel who require frequent contact spread throughout a building, poor communication networks can develop, resulting in role ambiguity and poor relationships. This problem is not restricted to offices. For example, one company found it had a high turnover of staff and absenteeism among its mainly female assembly line workers. When researchers looked into the problem, it was discovered that the women were isolated from each other due to the layout of conveyor belts used in the work. They felt bored and lonely working without human interaction. Once the assembly line was reorganized to put the women into groups, the absenteeism dropped substantially.

Shift Work

Many workers today have jobs requiring them to work in shifts, some of which involve working staggered hours. Studies have found that shift work is a common occupational stress factor. It has even been determined that shift work affects blood temperature, metabolic rate, blood sugar levels, mental efficiency and work motivation, not to mention sleep patterns and family and social life. In one study of air traffic controllers, shift work was isolated as a major problem area, although other major job stress agents were also present.[11] These workers had four times the prevalence of hypertension, and also more mild diabetes and peptic ulcers than did a control group of US Air Force personnel.

In a study of offshore oil rig workers, the third most important source of stress found was a general category labelled 'work patterns', such as shift work, physical conditions and travel.[12] The longer the work shift, for example 'twenty-eight days on, twenty-eight days off' versus 'fourteen days on, fourteen days off', the greater the stress. The shift work patterns were a predictor of mental and physical ill health, particularly when the oil rig workers were married and had children.

A major study of American nurses conducted by the Stanford Research Institute identified shift work as a major problem.[13] The study, which compared nurses working fixed shifts with those working rotating shifts, found that the rotating nurses fared the worst, followed closely by night-shift workers. Overall, these two groups tended to have 'more frequent and more serious physical complaints, more digestive problems and menstrual difficulties'. Shift rotators also reported a greater use of alcohol, a higher frequency of problems with their sex lives, and less satisfaction in their personal lives than other shift workers. Rotating shift nurses were significantly more confused, depressed and anxious than those nurses on non-rotating shifts. The investigators concluded that 'rotation was a scheduling system that imposes excessive physical and psychological costs to the workers'. The study also found that, unlike fixed-shift workers, those on rotating shifts showed little or no tendency to adapt over time.

As a positive note, researcher Hans Selye concluded that most investigators agree that shift work becomes physically less stressful as individuals can (and often do) adapt to the situation.

Long Hours

The long working hours required by many jobs appear to take a toll on employee health. One research study has made a link between long working hours and deaths due to coronary heart disease.[14] This investigation of light industrial workers in the US found that individuals under forty-five years of age who worked more than forty-eight hours a week, had twice the risk of death from coronary heart disease than did similar individuals working a maximum of forty hours a week.

Another study of 100 young coronary patients revealed that 25 per cent of them had been working at two jobs, and an additional 40 per cent worked for more than sixty hours a week.[15] Many individuals, such as executives working long hours and medical residents who might have no sleep for thirty-six hours or more, may find that both they, and the quality of their work, suffers. It is now commonly recognized that working beyond forty hours a week results in time spent that is increasingly unproductive.

THE STRESS OF NOT DELEGATING

'No, I don't find it easy to delegate, it's a major weakness of mine. In fact that's one of my stress points, in that I'd rather do it myself when somebody else could do it. An example recently springs to mind. I'm organizing a trip to France, which

I do every year, and I'd rather collect the money than let someone else do it. It's not that I don't trust other people, it's just that I'd rather keep tabs on it all the time so I know exactly what's going on. Maybe it has to do with the fact that I'll get blamed if something goes wrong.'

Travel

Although travel opportunities are an appealing bonus for many workers, travel can be a source of stress. Traffic jams on the road or at airports, delayed flights or trains, and the difficulties in the face of unknown places and people can present stress factors as well as challenges. Marriages and families may suffer if one member spends significant time away. In addition, a travelling worker spends less time with fellow workers and may miss out on opportunities or feel out of step with 'office politics'.

A SIGN OF COMMITMENT

'I'm not a great traveller. Although I like seeing places and new things, I don't particularly like business travelling because I find it a bit unsatisfactory – I only see the office and the hotel room, therefore I tend not to travel as much as I should. Some people do too much, they could use the telephone instead. There is a bit of company pressure sometimes, if I don't show myself keen to go, it might be thought you're disinterested. I'm prepared to be thought unkeen these days for the sake of my family. It is sometimes better to meet people face-to-face, but trips should be entered into judicially.'

Risk and Danger

As we saw in the stress league table, a job which involves risk or danger can result in higher stress levels. When someone is constantly aware of potential danger, he or she is prepared to react immediately. The individual is in a constant state of arousal, as described in the 'fight or flight' syndrome. The resulting adrenalin rush, respiration changes and muscle tension are all seen as potentially threatening to long-term health. On the other hand, individuals who face physical danger – such as policemen, mine workers, firemen and soldiers – often appear to have reduced stress levels, particularly those who are adequately trained and equipped to deal with emergency situations.

New Technology

The introduction of new technology into the work environment has required workers, particularly blue-collar workers, to continually adapt to new equipment, systems and ways of working. Having a boss trained in the 'old ways' may be an extra burden for the new employee trained in the latest methods, and raises questions about the adequacy of supervision and doubts of employees about those in senior positions.

In a study conducted by Cary Cooper of sources of stress among executives in ten countries, Japanese executives suffered particularly from pressure to 'keep up with new technology', that is, to maintain their technological superiority.[16] Managers in 'developing countries' feel pressure due to the increasing emphasis on new technology, the need to deal with an inadequately trained workforce and the imposition of deadlines. Also, in Britain, a high percentage of managers (second only to Japan) say that 'keeping up with new technology' is a great source of pressure at work. This is not surprising in a nation that many people feel is beginning to slip behind competitors in the race to grab new export markets. In addition, these British managers describe a high level of stress due to the 'amount of travel' required by their work.

Work Overload

Two different types of work overload have been described by researchers. 'Quantitative' overload refers simply to having too much work to do. 'Qualitative' overload refers to work that is too difficult for an individual.[17] In the first case, too much work often leads to working long hours, with the attendant problems described above. A too heavy work burden has also been connected with increased cigarette smoking.

In a 1973 study, twenty-two white-collar workers were observed for two or three hours a day for three days.[18] Two observers recorded data on events occurring in the job environment, and heart rate responses to these events. The workers also wore pocket-sized devices which assessed their heart rates without interfering with the workers' activities. The workers also filled out questionnaires describing their work load over the three-day period. The researchers found that those people who admitted to feeling work pressure were observed to suffer more interruptions from visitors and phone calls. Secondly, these workers suffered significantly more physiological strain through higher heart rates and higher cholesterol levels.

CONTROL

'I tend to work longer hours and sometimes that is counter-productive. I find that half of the time I don't overwork and half of the time I get sufficiently anxious to allow it to erode my personal and social life. It's very much to do with pressures over which you have very little control, control is a major issue relating to stress. I think for management it is the speed factor which is the big stress.'

Work Underload

Psychologist Tom Cox has described the problem of not being sufficiently challenged by work: 'Job underload associated with repetitive routine, boring and understimulating work has been associated with ill health.'[19] As Bob Slocum, the main character in Joseph Heller's novel *Something Happened!*, laments, 'I am bored with my work very often now. Everything that comes in I pass along to somebody else. This makes my boredom worse. It's a real problem to decide whether it's more boring to do something boring than to pass along everything that comes in to somebody else and then have nothing to do at all.'[20]

Certain workers, such as pilots, air traffic controllers, nuclear power workers, face a special aspect of work underload. They must deal with long periods of time in which they have little to do, facing the possibility that they may suddenly be required to spring into action in a crisis.

ROLE IN THE ORGANIZATION

When a person's role in an organization is clearly defined and understood, and when expectations placed upon the individual are also clear and non-conflicting, stress can be kept to a minimum. But as researchers have clearly seen, this is not the case in many worksites. Three critical factors, role ambiguity, role conflict and the degree of responsibility for others, are seen to be major sources of stress. Much of the research in this area has been carried out by the Survey Research Center of the University of Michigan.

Role Ambiguity

Role ambiguity arises when an individual does not have a clear picture about his work objectives, his co-workers' expectations of him, and the scope and responsibilities of his job. Often this ambiguity results simply because a supervisor does not lay out to the employee exactly what his role is. As Leon Warshaw states, 'The individual just doesn't know how he or she fits into the organization and is unsure of any rewards no matter how well he or she may perform.'[21]

There is a wide range of activities which can create role ambiguity. Ivancevich and Matteson highlight these: 'The first job, a promotion or transfer, a new boss, the first supervisory responsibility, a new company, or a change in the structure of the existing organization – all of these events and others, may serve to create a temporary state of role ambiguity.'[22]

The stress indicators found to relate to role ambiguity are depressed mood, lowered self-esteem, life dissatisfaction, low motivation to work and the intention to leave a job.

Role Conflict

Role conflict exists when an individual is torn by conflicting

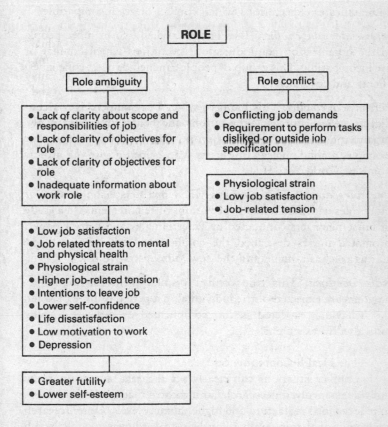

Figure 3. Sources of Role Stress at Work

job demands or by doing things he or she does not really want to do, or things which the individual does not believe are part of the job. Workers may often feel themselves torn between two groups of people who demand different types of behaviour or who believe the job entails different functions.

Quick and Quick [23] have described the following types of role conflict:

Intrasender role conflict: This happens when a boss or supervisor communicates expectations which conflict or are incompatible.

Intersender role conflict: This happens when two or more people in the organization communicate expectations which conflict or are incompatible. This group of people can include boss, colleagues, clients and customers.

Person role conflict: This happens when a person perceives a conflict between his or her expectations and beliefs and those of the organization or key people at work. Such a conflict arose, for example, among nuclear physicists who helped devise the atomic bomb in World War II.

Interrole conflict: This happens when one person holds two or more roles with conflicting expectations or requirements. In a study of nurse managers conducted by Peter Hingley and Cary Cooper, promoted nurses described the conflict they felt between their 'caring role' as a nurse and the new 'administrative role'.[24]

Role Overload: This role conflict results when 'too many behaviours are expected of the individual in a period of time or when the behaviour expected is too complicated or difficult for the individual to execute'.[25]

The Health Consequences

Conflict situations can clearly act as stress factors upon the individuals involved. Research has indicated that role conflict leads to reduced job satisfaction and higher anxiety levels. Other research has shown that role conflict can lead to cardiovascular ill health risks, such as elevated blood pressure, abnormal blood chemistry and so forth.[26]

One study of American dentists conducted by Cary Cooper, Mark Mallinger and Richard Kahn found that among the best predictors of abnormally high blood pressure levels among the dentists sampled were factors associated with the individuals' professional roles.[27] A high level of conflict was found between the idealized 'caring/healing' role and the actual reality of being 'an inflictor of pain'. In addition, the carrying out of administrative tasks and building up a practice, clashed with the commitment to a 'caring profession'.

Personality Variables

As might be expected, studies have shown that people with high anxiety levels suffer more from role conflicts than do people who are more flexible in their approach to life. As psychologists Peter Warr and Toby Wall of Sheffield University describe it: 'Anxiety prone individuals experienced role conflict more acutely and reacted to it with greater tension than did people who were less anxiety prone; and more flexible individuals responded to high role conflict with lesser feeling of tension than did their more rigid counterparts.'[28] In other studies, when the individual has stronger needs for cognitive clarity or lower levels of tolerance for ambiguity, job-related stress was found to be higher and more prolonged.

Responsibility

Responsibility has been found to be another organizational role stress agent. In an organization, there are basically two types of responsibility: responsibility for people, and responsibility for things, such as budgets, equipment and buildings. Responsibility for people has been found to be particularly stressful. Studies in the 1960s found that this was far more likely to lead to coronary heart disease than was responsibility for things.[29] Being responsible for people usually requires spending more time interacting with others, attending meetings and attempting to meet deadlines. An investigation in the United Kingdom of 1,200 managers sent by their companies for annual medical examinations linked physical stress to age and level of responsibility.[30] The older the executive and the more responsibility held by the executive, the greater the probability of coronary heart disease risk factors.

As Ivancevich and Matteson state, 'Part of the reason responsibility for people acts as a stressor undoubtedly results from

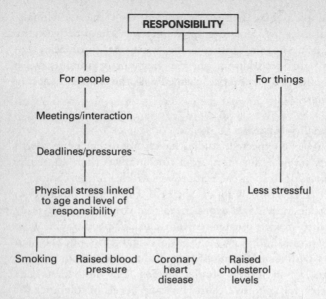

Figure 4. The Stress of Job Responsibility

the specific nature of the responsibility, particularly as it relates to the need to make unpleasant interpersonal decisions. Another part of the reason, as alluded to above, is that people in responsibility positions lend themselves to overload, and perhaps role conflict and ambiguity as well.'[31]

The stressful nature of having responsibility for others has grown in the economic climate of the 1980s, with so many industries facing decline. As industries implement cutbacks in production and sales, managers are caught between the two goals of 'keeping personnel costs to a minimum', while also looking after the 'welfare of subordinates' in terms of job security and stability.

In a study of an American police force, the responsibility for people and their safety was seen as a potentially significant occupational source of stress.[32] Another conducted by University of Manchester researchers isolated 'responsibility for people's safety and lives' as a major stress factor in predicting risk of heart disease among air traffic controllers.[33]

Other Organizational Role Factors

One role which has been seen to be particularly vulnerable to stress agents is that of 'middle manager'. Middle managers feel caught between the higher levels of command and the young new recruits. Middle managers often feel they have little real power and may feel vulnerable to redundancy or forced early retirement. Joseph Heller's *Something Happened!* includes a description which may match what many middle managers feel:

> What would happen, if, deliberately, calmly, with malice afore-thought and obvious premeditation, I disobeyed? I know what would happen: nothing. Nothing would happen. And the knowledge depresses me ... I suppose it is just about impossible for someone like me to rebel anymore and produce any kind of lasting effect. I have lost the power to upset things that I had as a child. I can no longer change my environment or even disturb it seriously. They would simply fire me and forget me as soon as I tried.

RELATIONSHIPS AT WORK

Other people – and our varied encounters with them – can be major sources of both stress and support. At work, especially, dealings with bosses, peers and subordinates can dramatically affect the way we feel at the end of the day. Stress researcher Hans Selye suggested that learning to live with other people is one of the most stressful aspects of life: 'good relationships between members of a group are a key factor in individual and organizational health'.[34]

It is an interesting fact, however, that little research has been done in this area. In 1966 Richard Lazarus suggested that supportive social relationships with peers, supervisors and subordinates at work are less likely to create interpersonal pressures, and will directly reduce levels of perceived job stress.[35] Poor relationships were defined by University of Michigan researchers as 'those which include low trust, low supportiveness, and low interest in listening and trying to deal with problems that confront the organizational member'.

Most studies have concluded that mistrust of fellow workers is connected with high role ambiguity, poor communications, and to 'psychological strain in the form of low job satisfaction and to

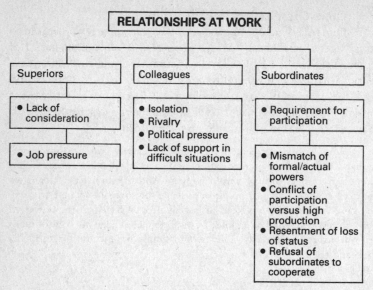

Figure 5. Stressful Relationships at Work

feelings of job-related threat to one's well being'.[36] Again, Joseph Heller humorously illustrates this concern about work relationships: 'In my department, there are six people who are afraid of me, and one small secretary who is afraid of all of us. I have one other person working for me who is not afraid of anyone, not even me, and I would fire him quickly, but I'm afraid of him.'

There are three critical relationships at work: relationships with superiors, relationships with subordinates and relationships with colleagues or co-workers.

Relationships with Superiors

Physicians and clinical psychologists support the idea that problems of emotional disability often result when the relationship between a subordinate and a boss is psychologically unhealthy for one reason or another. A 1972 study which focused on the relationship of workers to an immediate boss found that when the boss was perceived as 'considerate', there was 'friendship, mutual trust, respect and a certain warmth between boss and subordinate'.[37]

Workers who said their boss was low on consideration reported feeling more job pressure. Workers who were under pressure reported that their bosses did not give them criticism in a helpful way, played favourites and 'pulled rank and took advantage of them whenever they had got a chance'.

Relationships with Subordinates

The way in which a manager supervises the work of others has always been considered a critical aspect of his or her work. For instance, the 'inability to delegate' has been a common criticism levelled against some managers. It now appears that managers face a new challenge: learning to govern by *participation*. Today's emphasis on participation can be a cause of resentment, anxiety, and stress for the managers involved. Researchers Dan Gower and Karen Legge[38] point to the factors which can make participatory management difficult:

1 Mismatch of formal and actual powers.
2 Managers' resentment of the erosion of formal roles and powers.
3 Pressure to be both participative and to meet high production standards.
4 Subordinates' refusal to participate.

Managerial stress may be particularly high for those individuals with technical and scientific backgrounds, which may be more 'things-orientated'. For these managers, personal relationships may appear more 'trivial' and 'time-consuming' than for managers who concern themselves with people. Cary Cooper and Judi Marshall found this to be particularly true among research and development scientists who had been promoted to management jobs.[39] Individuals promoted to management positions on the basis of their technical skills, without management training, often encounter serious relationship problems at work.

Relationships with Colleagues

Stress among co-workers can arise from the competition and personality conflicts usually described as 'office politics'. As we discussed in Chapter 3, adequate social support can be critical to the health and well-being of an individual and to the atmosphere and success of an organization. Because most people spend so much time at work, the relationships among co-workers can provide valuable support or, conversely, can be a huge source of stress. University of Michigan researchers found that strong social support from co-workers eased job strain. This support also mediated the effects of job strain on cortisone levels, blood pressure, glucose levels, and the number of cigarettes smoked.[40]

Many high-ranking executives appear to suffer from the *lack* of a peer group, rather than from actual negative interaction. In a highly competitive environment, problem-solving may be inhibited because managers do not want to appear weak. Once again, Bob Slocum in *Something Happened!* reflects: 'I always feel very secure and very superior when I'm sitting inside someone's office with the door closed and other people, perhaps Kagle, or Green or Brown, are doing all the worrying on the outside about what's going on, in the inside.'

Interpersonal Demands

In the preceding section, we examined the three major types of personal relationships that are faced at work and the stress they can create. Behavioural scientists Quick and Quick have designed another way of looking at stress agents which arise from social relationships at work.[41] They define five types of 'interpersonal stressors', which result from the demands and pressures of work relationships. These are:

1 Status incongruence
2 Social density
3 Abrasive personalities
4 Leadership style
5 Group pressures

Status Incongruence

Quick and Quick state that 'each individual occupies a unique social status within a group within an organization, which is based on a range of factors such as education, income, family background, socio-economic class, and so on. Many people within an organization often feel they do not have as much power, influence and prestige as they deserve. This feeling can cause enormous frustration and resentment in the workplace.

Restricted job opportunities in many industries can thwart individual ambition and can leave many managers feeling 'trapped'. This frustration can be directed towards the organization or an authority figure within it. Heller highlights this problem in *Something Happened!*:

Green is a clever tactician with long experience at office politics. He is a talented, articulate, intelligent man of fifty-six and has been with the company more than thirty years. He was a young man when he came here; he will soon be old. He has longed from the beginning to become a Vice President and now knows that he will never succeed . . . He continues to yearn and he continues to strive and scheme, sometimes cunningly, other times desperately, abjectly, ineptly, because he can neither admit nor deny to himself for very long that he has already failed.

On the other hand, when a person is promoted or put into a role of higher status than he or she is used to, a feeling of insecurity can result. This individual may feel he or she lacks the necessary social skills to 'fit in' and may feel under undue scrutiny. For example, Bob Slocum in *Something Happened!* characterizes fellow worker Andy Kagle: 'Kagle is not comfortable with people on his own level or higher. He tends to sweat on his forehead and upper lip, and to bubble in the corners of his mouth. He feels he doesn't belong with them.'

Social Density

Each person desires his own amount of 'personal space'; some people will feel uncomfortable when working too near others, while others will feel isolated if they are not near fellow workers. In a study of international interpreters by Rachel and Cary Cooper, it was found that sharing an 'interpreting booth' with an incompatible colleague was a major source of job dissatisfaction and lack of mental well-being.[42] Situations which crowd many people together for long periods of time, such as accommodation for offshore oil rig workers, will prove to be stressful for those who need substantial personal space. On the other hand, those who are stimulated by so much contact with others, may actually enjoy the closeness.

For many women, the decision to return to work after the birth of a child is influenced greatly by the desire to be around other adults. Also, people working on their own often feel the need to be with others. For example, a British company was formed to provide 'home-based' computer programming for working mothers. After a period of time, it was discovered that the women's need for social contact necessitated regional offices and more meetings of the house-bound programmers.

Abrasive Personalities

A particular personality – that of the abrasive, hard-driving, achievement-orientated individual – has been seen to create stress for those around him or her. Harry Levinson states that these abrasive people cause stress for other individuals because they find no time to consider working relationships and ignore the interpersonal aspects of feelings and sensibilities within social interaction.[43]

Leadership Style

The potential stress for individuals exposed to an authoritarian leadership style is well documented.[44] There is a delicate balance between stimulating subordinates towards growth and development, and creating a negative environment of hostility and pressure. The deterioration in working relationships between a boss and subordinates can lead to disrupted working relationships, reduced well-being, high blood pressure levels and reduced safety consciousness.

Group Pressures

Both formal and informal groups within an organization can exert pressure upon individuals, often creating a source of stress at work. As Quick and Quick state: 'As a group matures through its developmental stages, it establishes a variety of behavioral norms which function as standards of conduct for members of the group. These behavioral norms are frequently unwritten and operate through a process of consensual understanding.' The violation of such a norm 'typically results in group sanctions to realign the individual's behavior with the norms . . . the purpose of such group-sanctioning behavior is to establish control over individual group members. As such, it causes stress and tension for the individual involved.'[45]

Group pressures are often apparent in unwritten, unofficial 'dress codes' at work. For example, one young professional woman hired at a major US accounting firm was the target of subtle ridicule from co-workers because she wore a tailored flannel hat with her winter coat. When she persisted in wearing the hat to and from work, she eventually received word from a manager, that a partner had decreed she leave the hat at home. One irony of the situation was that until a few years before the woman's hiring, female professionals at the firm were required to wear hats.

Informal groups at work can also influence the amount of work performed. Eager young recruits who are willing to push themselves to the limit are often 'brought into line' by more experienced workers who do not want management's expectations about production levels to be raised.

CAREER DEVELOPMENT

A host of issues can act as potential stress factors throughout one's working life. The lack of job security; fear of redundancy, obsolescence or retirement; and numerous performance appraisals can cause pressure and strain. In addition, as we have already examined, the frustration of having reached one's career ceiling, or having been over-promoted can result in extreme stress. Ivancevich and Matteson suggest that individuals suffering from 'career stress' often show high job dissatisfaction, job mobility, burnout, poor work performance, less effective interpersonal relationships at work, and so on.[46]

Job Security

For many workers, career progression is of overriding importance – by promotion, people earn not only money, but enjoy increased status and new challenges. In the early years at a job, the striving and ability required to deal with a rapidly changing

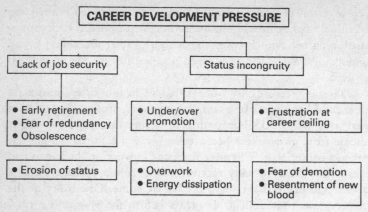

Figure 6. Career Stresses

environment is usually rewarded by a company through monetary and promotional rewards. At middle age, however, many people find their career progress has slowed or stopped. Job opportunities may become fewer, available jobs can require longer to master, old knowledge may become obsolete, and energy levels can flag at the same time 'younger' competition threatens.

FEAR OF JOB LOSS AND THE HEART

'My husband is very fond of his company, he's a company man, so when the company was in a bit of trouble and he thought he might lose his job, he suffered greatly. At first he showed it in agitation with me and the children, but finally in a heart attack. In a way the heart attack was quite a relief, it forced my husband to put his job and life into perspective and he has been able to cope with both much better. The fear of losing a job, though, can really damage your self-confidence and family life. I speak from experience!'

The fear of demotion or obsolescence can be strong for those who believe they will suffer some erosion of status before they retire. Heller's character Bob Slocum illustrates this experience:

People in the company are almost never fired; if they grow inadequate or obsolete ahead of schedule, they are encouraged to retire early or are eased aside into hollow, insignificant, newly created positions with fake functions and no authority, where they are sheepish and unhappy for as long as they remain; nearly always they must occupy a small and less convenient office, sometimes one with another person already in it; or, if they are still young, they're simply encouraged directly (although with courtesy) to find better jobs with other companies and then resign.

The Older Worker and Retirement

One's last years at a job may provide particular strains and pressures. Studies by Ann McGoldrick and Cary Cooper have shown a widespread awareness of these pressures in the later years at work, pressures which become more significant with increasing age of employees.[47] A survey of 1,200 workers facing early retirement showed the majority became less satisfied with their jobs in the years before retirement, and about half experienced changing attitudes towards their work and found their jobs harder to cope with.

The transition to retirement can be in itself a stressful event. While a job is a socially defined role, retirement has been described as the 'roleless role'.[48] The vagueness and lack of structure of retirement can provide problems for the ill-prepared. For some individuals, becoming 'pensioners' or 'senior citizens' presents a situation in which they are uncertain how to obtain the social rewards they value. In contrast, those individuals who have maintained balance in their lives by developing interests and friends outside their work can find retirement a liberating period.

Job Performance

The process of being evaluated and appraised can be a stressful experience for all of us. It must be recognized that performance appraisals can be anxiety provoking, for both the individual being examined and the person doing the judging and appraising. The supervisor making performance judgements faces the threat of union grievance procedures in some cases, as well as interpersonal strains and the responsibility of making decisions affecting another's person's livelihood.

The way in which an evaluation is carried out can affect the degree of anxiety experienced. For example, taking a written examination can be a short-term stress factor, while continuous and confidential appraisals by supervisors can have a more long-term effect, depending on the structure and climate of the organization.

ORGANIZATIONAL STRUCTURE AND CLIMATE

Just being part of an organization can present threats to an individual's sense of freedom and autonomy. Organizational workers sometimes complain they do not have a sense of belonging, lack adequate opportunities to participate, feel their behaviour is unduly restricted and are not included in office communications and consultations.

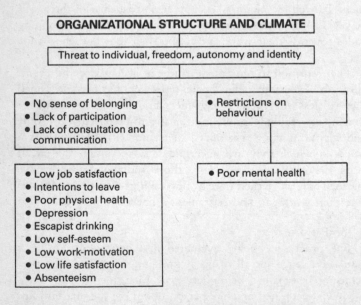

Figure 7. The Stress of the Organizational Environment

Participation at Work

As early as the 1940s, researchers began reporting that workers who were allowed more participation in decision-making produced more and had higher job satisfaction.[49] They also found that non-participation at work was a significant predictor of strain and job-related stress, relating to general poor health, escapist drinking, depression, low self-esteem, absenteeism and plans to leave work.[50] Participation in the decision-making process on the part of the individual may help increase his feeling of investment in the company's success, create a sense of belonging and improve communication channels within the organization. The resulting sense of being in control seems vital for the well-being of the work-force.

AUTONOMY AT WORK

'I like the day-to-day work with the organization and the people, it's nice to be needed. There's a very obvious need for the job to exist, therefore it feels worthwhile. I have to be honest and say I enjoy the power and influence I am able to exert. I enjoy being the centre of things and that fills a lot of my personal needs, being active and knowing what is going on. Also I like accomplishing things and seeing the ends of my work. I also enjoy freedom to act on my own . . . there aren't many rules as to how the job's to be done and this gives me satisfaction.'

A major commitment to worker participation has been made at the Volvo automobile assembly plants. At the Kalmar plant in Sweden, Volvo has launched its most famous and daring partici-pation effort. Workers rotate jobs and work towards a quota set by the planning department and the union. No overtime is paid for working extra hours. Employees work until the quota is met and then have free time. If they finish early, they may take a sauna or swim at the plant. Workers elect their own supervisors, who are paid a slightly higher rate and can be replaced by a vote at any time. Replacement workers are brought in at the group's consent and are trained by the group. Job sharing is widely practised, with two people, often a husband and wife, splitting the shift or working alternate days. A spirit of co-operation and fair play, essential to a worker participation plan, seems in good evidence at Volvo.

Industrial Relations

The current climate in many organizations appears to be characterized by growing rigidity in management and worker roles, lack of understanding and communication between those in the two different roles, and lack of genuine efforts at long-term resolution of problems. Repeated confrontations can only damage the organizational climate, reducing trust and encouraging workers and managers to blame one another for their deteriorating standards of living.

STRESSFUL EVENTS AT WORK

Sudden changes in the work environment can prove stressful for certain individuals, especially those who do not feel confident in their ability to deal with change. Major company decisions, such as the closing of a division or plant site, the relocation of a group of employees, or a reduction in the size of the work force can prove tremendously stressful. As with any stressful event, however, the individual personality, coping style and support can make a large difference in the amount of threat perceived and how a person responds to it.

STRESSFUL LIFE EVENT

Mr Clark is forty-seven and a senior manager with a printing firm. When he was recruited to the research project several years ago his medical examination proved normal. Then two years ago his smaller firm was taken over by a larger printing firm and his future became doubtful. He began to have frequent episodes of panic, in which he was very conscious of his heart beat, began to sweat profusely and was fearful of crowded places.

After the takeover, he found his job was retained and his future more secure. The episodes of panic evaporated until a year later when he was up for promotion. He and a close colleague were competing for the same senior post and during this period Mr Clark found himself once again experiencing palpitations of the heart, frequent episodes of panic, sweating and tear of crowds.

He had to take two weeks off work due to 'nervous debility' and had to be driven to work by a chauffeur or colleague for the next four weeks. His inability to cope with the situation at work fed back into his home life and created difficulties as well. This circular process of pressure at work affecting personal relationships at home, and then adverse home life affecting work performance, is a typical problem affecting the well-being of the executive.

PERSON–ENVIRONMENT FIT

In Chapter 1 we outlined the stress model which emphasizes the crucial interaction between an individual and his environment. When looking more specifically at the fit between a person and his work environment, it is important to keep in mind the individual nature of the stress response. Matching a person to his or her environment at work can be defined as an interaction between an individual's psychological and social characteristics and objective work conditions. Looking at the first factor, it can be noted that there are some individuals who seem by nature to be excessively vulnerable and who have difficulty coping with even relatively mundane tasks; for them personality variables will always dominate the stress equation.

In other instances, the work situation or environment may be entirely to blame. And, of course, a work situation which one individual finds stressful, another person will find stimulating and satisfying. Further complicating the picture is the realization that some individuals can find their job so satisfying that they over-invest their time and energy in it, putting health and social life in jeopardy. Here we see the necessity of balance, as discussed earlier.

An interesting study of work stress conducted by University of Michigan researchers looked at how people with either introverted or extroverted personalities react to stressful events at work.[51] It was found, for example, that when an introverted person is under stress from role conflict, he will tend to reduce contacts with other people. This defensive withdrawal aggravates those attempting to define his role, causing them to view the introvert as too independent. These 'role senders' will intensify their efforts to influence him, putting him under increased interpersonal pressure. The introvert's coping strategy can prove self-defeating.

The extrovert, on the other hand, is not as open to role conflict as the introvert, and will usually react more openly and adaptively if it does occur. The different ways in which extroverts and introverts deal with role conflict can play a significant part in determining the 'fit' between individuals and their jobs. An introvert, for instance, could be expected to be more comfortable in a clearly defined role, where conflicting expectations are held to a minimum.

The Michigan researchers also compared rigid and flexible personality types. They found that rigid people tend to avoid conflict, showing increased dependence on authority figures and relying on compulsive work habits. By reacting in this way, the rigid person avoids the immediate conflict, but further isolates himself from the reality of the situation. Flexible people show more varied responses to pressure, responding primarily by complying with work demands and seeking support from peers and subordinates. The compliance can lead to work overload problems, while the reliance on those of equal and lower rank does not involve those most able to help, that is, those superiors setting out work expectations. It can be seen that the responses of both the rigid and flexible personality types can create potential problems. It is clear, however, that different personality types will be more suitable for particular jobs than others. For example, the rigid individual will be at risk in a situation which requires him to adapt and cope with a fast-changing environment.

WORK STRESS ACROSS CULTURES

The kind of job stress experienced by individuals will vary according to their culture. Significant differences have been seen between developed and developing countries in terms of job satisfaction, mental well-being and sources of job stress. In a study by Cary Cooper of nearly 1,100 senior to top-level executives in ten countries, it was found that each country presents its own idiosyncratic work pressures.[52] For instance, US executives perceive their greatest sources of pressure at work to be 'lack of power and influence', 'incompetent bosses', and 'beliefs conflicting with those of the organization'. In contrast, Japanese executives, more than any other country's executives, rated 'keeping up with new technology' as a major source of strain and job dissatisfaction. Swedish executives most often cited stresses involving the encroachment of work upon their private lives. Germans complained of 'time pressures' and 'working with inadequately trained subordinates'. South African executives as well complained of 'inadequately trained subordinates'.

In Singapore, where entrepreneurial values of the West are prevalent, executives seem to suffer most of their stress at work from an inability to transmit their own ambitions or skills to those below them. Nigerian executives show strains of having to perform in a rapidly growing economy, with lack of a properly developed management infrastructure. They complain about inadequately trained subordinates, long working hours and 'doing a job below my level of competence'. In Brazil, executives appear under extreme pressure, as reflected in very high mental ill health and job dissatisfaction. Stresses affecting performance range from time pressures, keeping up with new technology, performing below competence levels and coping with inadequately trained personnel. In Egypt, it appears a wide range of stress factors adversely affect executives: work overload, inadequately trained subordinates, and taking work home. Other problems mentioned in the study reflect an overload of bureaucracy.

As the study reflects, each culture, like each organization, produces its unique set of job satisfactions and pressures. Those individuals responsible for the well-being of managers and other employees must be cognizant of these factors.

Table 2. Sources of Executive Stress (% of respondents)

Which of the following are a source of pressure for you at work?	Britain	Sweden	Germany	Japan
Time pressures and deadlines	61.5	53.8	65.4	41.8
Work overload	57.3	55.9	59.1	41.8
Amount of travel required by my work	61.1	20.0	18.2	18.7
Long working hours	26.6	33.8	27.3	26.1
Taking my work home	17.5	29.6	16.4	13.4
Lack of power and influence	20.3	11.0	19.1	17.9
Attending meetings	21.7	21.4	23.6	20.9
My beliefs conflicting with those of the organization	20.3	14.5	21.8	20.1
Keeping up with new technology	25.9	19.3	14.5	32.8
Doing a job below the level of my competence	13.3	10.3	20.0	18.7
Inadequately trained subordinates	13.1	20.0	26.4	24.6
Interpersonal relations	15.4	14.5	15.4	29.8
Demands of work on my relationship with my family	22.4	26.9	25.4	11.2
Demands on my private and social life	18.2	31.7	19.1	14.9
Incompetent boss	9.1	11.7	19.1	13.4

Totals do not add to 100 per cent because of multiple answers.

Singapore	US	Nigeria	S. Africa	Brazil	Egypt	Total
55.3	46.5	54.0	59.1	61.8	45.0	55.3
44.7	53.5	50.4	48.2	30.1	76.7	51.6
20.0	16.3	29.7	16.8	9.3	16.7	18.4
22.3	30.2	40.5	34.3	19.6	23.3	29.0
15.3	27.9	19.8	19.0	15.5	30.0	19.7
22.3	46.5	20.7	22.6	18.5	11.7	19.5
25.9	16.3	25.2	28.5	27.8	20.0	23.6
21.2	30.2	26.1	24.8	16.5	13.3	20.6
20.0	13.9	18.0	21.9	24.7	10.0	21.4
12.9	18.6	23.4	20.4	23.7	20.0	17.7
47.0	25.5	56.7	36.5	41.2	65.0	36.4
12.9	13.9	16.2	24.1	25.8	23.3	19.4
12.9	16.3	29.7	29.2	8.2	25.0	21.4
12.9	16.3	30.6	29.9	13.4	26.7	22.1
16.5	30.2	18.0	16.1	16.5	20.0	15.6

SPECIAL STRESS FACTORS FOR WOMEN AT WORK

For women at work, the stress equation takes on additional complexities, both in terms of the personality side of the equation and the environmental conditions to be faced.[53] A number of causes of stress can arise from 'within the woman' herself. Many women, taking on management positions in particular, may discover conflicts within themselves. It is obvious that a great deal of learning about sex-roles takes place among women during the early phases of their lives, and this can translate itself into an attitude of mind that creates difficulties later in work life or life generally. Laurie Larwood and Marion Wood in their book *Women in Management* describe internal blocks that women experience which derive from early sex stereotyping and socialization.[54] Firstly, many women are caught in a 'low expectation trap', particularly when performing a job usually done by men. Women can feel that their performance is unequal to the task. This feeling is often a self-fulfilling prophecy. Secondly, some theorists believe certain women fear success, and may avoid success in order to 'behave in a socially approved manner'.[55] This feeling can inhibit further effort and achievement. Thirdly, most women are not socialized to be assertive or aggressive or to seek power and control. As psychologist David McClelland has pointed out, the most successful male managers are the most assertive and have the most highly developed desire for power.[56] Women would, therefore, seem disadvantaged from their 'pink' cradle of birth. It can be countered, however, that there is a different management style that is compatible with the more traditional, less aggressive, female role. Fourthly, many women have been expected and encouraged to be dependent upon men, a fact that some researchers believe makes women less self-reliant and more amenable to influence.

This 'culture trap' creates difficulties for working women because most organizations are dominated by male values and behaviours, while women are still encouraged to pay a less achievement-orientated, less aggressive, more dependent role. Perhaps, as women gain hold of more significant and powerful positions in

Sources of stress

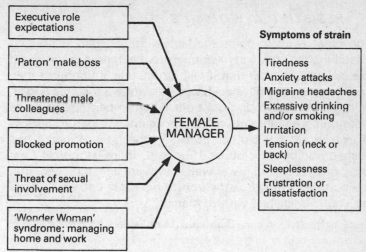

Figure 8: Stress and the Female Manager

industry, the more aggressive values of contemporary business will change, to be replaced by an amalgam of female and male values. In the meantime, however, women managers are at a disadvantage and are forced to use the behavioural armoury of their male associates to succeed. Some common stress factors faced by female managers and the resulting symptoms of strain are pointed out in Figure 8.

Executive Role Expectations

A major source of stress for career women derives from the concept of the professional woman held by themselves and others. While a man can suffer from lack of role clarity and role conflict, he does so because of his individual situation, not because he is a man. The same cannot be said of a woman attempting to fill a role previously held only by men. Self-doubt and concern about meeting other people's expectations must continually hover over the thoughts and actions of women managers.

RESISTING A 'WOMAN'S ROLE'

'I deliberately avoid doing the female things such as pouring or fetching the coffee at meetings, etc. I am often asked and if I do it, I make it clear that it will be the man's turn from then on. On occasions I have even said I do not want coffee and let them get their own and sat tight. I remember, also, on one occasion I went abroad with my boss and we had to borrow an iron to get our clothes ironed in the hotel. When I had finished ironing my clothes, I thought, there is no way I am going to offer to iron his as well – if I were a man he wouldn't expect it. So, I just took the iron to his room and said, "Here you are, I've finished with it, thanks."'

'Patron' Male Boss

While some male bosses may feel threatened by a young career woman who works doubly hard to prove herself, most research indicates that most men are supportive of their female subordinates. This especially holds true for a highly competent female subordinate who does not threaten her boss's relationship with male colleagues. The supportive male boss plays a 'patron' role, which holds potential strains of its own for the woman. The patron protects and advances his protégé, but at the same time uses her competence for his own advancement. Although this shielding and advancement has definite advantages, it also holds built-in pressures. Firstly, the woman may feel she must always perform at her best to meet her patron's expectations. Secondly, she can identify with him and suffer the professional trials and tribulations that he experiences. Thirdly, significant people within the organization may not recognize her talents, which are always seen as fused with his. Fourthly, the career woman in this case is still playing a dependent role by not 'making a mark' based on her own resources. All these factors intertwine to create layers of expectations, which can place significant stress on the career woman.

Threat of Sexual Involvement

Sexuality at work is a double-edged sword for the working woman. On the one hand, she may experience the pressures of sexual harassment from men who hold the keys to her future success. On the other hand, a woman may utilize her sexual role to achieve career objectives, often resulting in unforeseen complications. Although there is little evidence that this manipulative sexual role is often played by career women, it is certain that both males and females can potentially use sexuality at work.

More often than not, the main stress factor a woman experiences as a result of an explicit sexual advance from a colleague involves the many issues surrounding the advance. Is he attracted to her physical attributes or her intellect and work capabilities? If he is interested in her as a woman, what does this mean to her about her skill, and about his professional attitude towards her? This conflict can present an enormous source of stress for women at the beginning of their careers, when they may lack self-confidence.

Threatened Male Colleague

Although many women claim they are helped by their male bosses, they often report that male colleagues of similar rank are excessively competitive, create stress for them and seem to be threatened by them. Some men at junior and middle management levels, for example, feel particularly threatened because they see their organizations promoting women as 'tokens' of equality. Male managers who are threatened by their female counterparts, for whatever reason, can and do create strains for women managers. This reaction can be as subtle as failing to provide complete information needed to make an important decision or by maintaining a distant and cool working relationship. It can be argued that this is common enough for men working together; why should women be shielded?

Blocked Promotion

Women struggling up the career ladder face obstacles at all levels, some of which involve the conflict between work and home. Many companies expect an employee to be willing to move for a job promotion or to take on short-term assignments away from home. Female managers with a family, for example, are unlikely to be able to do either, often appearing less of a 'company man' than their male counterparts.

The 'Wonder Woman' Syndrome

Most working women also have the responsibility for a home and family as well. Juggling a job and a family is often done at the expense of a woman's physical and psychological health. The dual-career family is becoming the norm, a fact that involves considerable strain for the women and men involved, as will be discussed in Chapter 5. Evidence that women are paying a price for the 'wonder woman' role appears in coronary heart disease figures. In a famous study of the population of a town called Framingham, the US National Heart, Lung and Blood Institute found that 'among working women the incidence of coronary heart disease rose as the number of children increased'.[57] This was not the case, however, for women who were exclusively homemakers. In fact, the homemaking group showed a slight decrease in heart disease with an increased number of children.

DIAGNOSING PROBLEMS

In this chapter numerous causes of work stress can be diagnosed. Organizations which have recognized such work stress problems often employ consultants to diagnose the causes and suggest means of reducing stress factors. Interviews, questionnaires and observation techniques are used to uncover causes of stress and it can also be helpful for an individual to diagnose his or her own sources of stress, such as extreme deadline pressure. The following work stress questionnaire can help you identify your particular work stressors (more detailed and comprehensive work questionnaires can be found in Cooper, Sloan and Williams[58]).

Chapter 6 will provide some guidance on how individuals and companies can cope with work stress. Before turning to solutions, however, we will examine the second major area of 'life stress', that is, stress outside of work.

Table 3. Cooper's Work Stress Questionnaire

Could you please circle the number that best reflects the degree to which the particular statement is a source of stress for you at work.

	No stress at all		Stress		A great deal of stress	
Work overload	0	1	2	3	4	5
Work underload	0	1	2	3	4	5
Time pressures and deadlines	0	1	2	3	4	5
The amount of travel required by my work	0	1	2	3	4	5
Long working hours	0	1	2	3	4	5
Taking my work home	0	1	2	3	4	5
Lack of power and influence	0	1	2	3	4	5
Attending meetings	0	1	2	3	4	5
My beliefs conflicting with those of the organization	0	1	2	3	4	5
Keeping up with new technology	0	1	2	3	4	5
Threat of job loss	0	1	2	3	4	5
Competition of promotion	0	1	2	3	4	5
Having to move with my job in order to progress my career	0	1	2	3	4	5
Doing a job beyond the level of my competence	0	1	2	3	4	5
Doing a job below the level of my competence	0	1	2	3	4	5
Inadequately trained subordinates	0	1	2	3	4	5
Interpersonal relations	0	1	2	3	4	5

Hiring and firing personnel	0	1	2 3	4 5
Unsympathetic boss	0	1	2 3	4 5
Incompetent boss	0	1	2 3	4 5
Performance-related compensation	0	1	2 3	4 5
Unrealistic objectives	0	1	2 3	4 5
Dealing with conservation groups	0	1	2 3	4 5
Dealing with shareholders	0	1	2 3	4 5
Dealing with unions	0	1	2 3	4 5
My spouse's attitude towards my career	0	1	2 3	4 5
Demands of work on my relationship with my family	0	1	2 3	4 5
Demands of work on private and social life	0	1	2 3	4 5
My relationship with my colleagues	0	1	2 3	4 5
My relationship with my subordinates	0	1	2 3	4 5
Making mistakes	0	1	2 3	4 5
Feeling undervalued	0	1	2 3	4 5
Promotion prospects	0	1	2 3	4 5
Rate of pay	0	1	2 3	4 5
Managing people	0	1	2 3	4 5
Office politics	0	1	2 3	4 5
Lack of consultation and communication in my organization	0	1	2 3	4 5

Chapter Five

SOURCES OF LIFE STRESS

> Oh, lift me as a wave, a leaf, a cloud!
> I fall upon the thorns of life! I bleed!
> Shelley

'Change is here to stay' is an old adage whose truth permeates all our lives. Change is, in fact, one of the monumental stress factors of our time. Alvin Toffler in *Future Shock* suggested that 'there are discoverable limits to the amount of change that the human organism can absorb . . . by endlessly accelerating these limits, we may submit masses of men to demands they simply cannot tolerate'.[1] Jack Ivancevich goes on to suggest that Toffler's depiction of change has been so rapid in Western society that one can look at it in terms of a series of lifetimes, 'dividing the past 50,000 years of human history into lifetimes of about sixty-two years gives us about 800 human lifetimes. The first 650 of these lifetimes were spent living in caves. Writing has been available only for the past seventy lifetimes, making it possible to preserve information from one lifetime to the next. The wide use of print has developed within the last 6 lifetimes. We have only been able to measure time with precision for about 4 lifetimes. The electric motor is a creature of the last 2 lifetimes.'[2]

Not only is there technological change, but also enormous social change in our lives, particularly in the role of women in society, a fact which has a major impact on marriage and child rearing. In addition, rising expectations of material and social success have created societal pressures and, often, disappointments, when expectations are not realized.

Besides the rapid societal change now confronting us, each of us must deal with a fairly predictable pattern of events and changes during a lifetime. At each stage of an individual's life cycle there are different sources of stress and satisfaction. In an effort to develop a clearer picture of these stress factors, we will look briefly at the early stages of childhood, adolescence and single adulthood, and then will examine in depth the later stages of marriage and parenting.

SOURCES OF STRESS DURING THE LIFE CYCLE

Childhood and Adolescence

Probably the most important time in our lives, even if a great deal of it is spent pre-consciously or only just consciously, is childhood. John Milton reflected this in his perceptive line, 'the childhood shows the man, as morning shows the day'. Childhood is a time of developing relationships, incessant learning, rewards and punishments, disappointments and achievements. It is above all about meeting one's own and other people's expectations.

Given the massive social and technological change, there is increasing pressure on adolescents to begin earlier to consider their future careers, and to continue with more and more education. This pressure has begun to reflect itself in drug and alcohol problems among adolescents, particularly in the developed countries of Western Europe and North America. Indeed, the most recent manifestations of this pressure, youth suicides in the United States (where it is now the second leading cause of death among teenagers) and in Japan (where it is now the leading cause of death among teenagers), and in other Western countries, is a worrying trend.

The leading sources of stress during this period seem to involve meeting the expectations of parents, teachers, peer groups, and the subculture. There are numerous books about this problem area and what can be done to manage the stresses involved. It is important to recognize that as the male and female roles in society undergo gradual but radical change, the problems experienced by young children and adolescents multiply.

Children are attempting to pinpoint and identify expectations in a constantly changing world, where parenting roles are in flux, where there is greater mobility (geographic and social), where there is less support, and where there are less clear role models of appropriate and inappropriate behaviour.

These problems do not stop at adolescence but multiply when one enters higher education. Take, for instance, a young female student in her first year at university, away from home for the first time. At school she did well, but now feels the pressure to continue this success. She finds the orientation towards self-discipline in her academic work difficult and the work more complex.

She spends most of her time studying, whereas her friends are having fun socializing. She worries about her methods of studying, her lecturers seem aloof and she is unable to ask for help. Having less and less confidence in her abilities, she works even harder.

She misses her parents and boyfriend, and finds it difficult to find the time to go home. In addition, she is having problems living on a grant and looking after herself. She has lost the comfortable social support of her home life and wonders if it is all worthwhile.[3]

Single Adult

The single person, in pursuit of his or her career, has a number of potential sources of stressors that can create difficulties, such as the culture shock of starting work after life at college, having no 'safe haven' of a family to offer support after work in the corporate jungle, and having difficulty making social contacts in a strange community (with mobility now being the rule rather than the exception in the workplace). Nevertheless, if he or she is geared towards career and achievement, the lateral and promotional moves should be of little social or psychological consequence. As long as the organization is aware of the performance and expectations of these young singles and rewards their efforts appropriately, the career plans made by the organization on their behalf should not create insurmountable difficulties. The two caveats, however, are important ones from the single adult's point of view. First, one must remember, these 'young singles' are at the 'adult mastery' stage of their development, that is, they are trying to prove themselves adults, not only to themselves but to others as well.[4] The application of reward systems is, therefore, critical for their continuing motivation and job satisfaction. In addition, it is important for management to take into account the expectations of young 'first entry' employees. All too often a conflict arises between high expectations and the actual experience of the job. This is due, in part, to management's lack of sensitivity to the potential of these new recruits or management's reluctance to take risks by delegating to them.

Many young adults are not only trying to find their work, but are also trying to answer personal questions, such as whether to marry. Both young men and young women are often faced with a decision of whether to marry before establishing themselves at a job, or delay marriage and family in order to concentrate on work. Single women especially may find the marriage issue difficult. Many cross-cultural studies have shown that female managers, for example, are only a third to a half likely to be married as male managers, and are less likely to have children. Certainly, unlike her married counterpart, a single woman limits the number of social roles she must play and the resulting degrees of role conflict. In fact, none of the twenty-five top US women managers interviewed by M. Henning and A. Jardim in their book *The Managerial Woman* were married or had chosen to have any significant personal life until their mid-thirties.[5] With respect to attitudes of organizations, the married males often tend to be viewed as an asset, whereas the married females are a liability.

Young single people living alone for the first time may experience the challenges and pressures of budgeting, establishing a home, and dealing with domestic details of shopping and laundry. Young bachelors may find it especially difficult to cope with these last necessities, although single women also describe the need for 'a wife' to take care of the home scene and provide emotional support. A female management trainee complained that, 'Unlike me, if the guys get married it wouldn't matter, as the company believes that men should have wives, and that it is an advantage, because if you move around a lot the wife can be the one looking after the children and buying the new house, while they are at work. I put it to them once that I didn't have a wife to do that for me, and therefore it makes life a bit difficult. Their reply was "hard cheese".'

It is common for single women in their late twenties to mention dilemmas relating to decisions on marriage and childbearing. A factory manager, who had climbed higher up the managerial ladder in her company than any other woman before her, related her career versus marriage conflict:

I would have been married by now if I hadn't been career-orientated. I wanted this job more than any of my other boyfriends and I have left them to move to my jobs. People say to me that if any of them had been 'Mr Right', I wouldn't have taken the jobs. I don't know but certainly the job seemed much more exciting at the time.

I'm twenty-six now and would like to think either this year or next, I will get a production manager job. However, I would like to get married and have a family and am worried as to how I'm going to manage it. One half of me wants to see myself as the efficient well-organized career woman who has two children and only takes a couple of months off work; the half of me which has been inbred in women for the last two and a half million years says I would like to be at home with my children and bring them up, and read lots of books on Freud. Three or four years ago if anyone suggested to me I was going to end up getting married and having children, I would have laughed at them. You're torn both ways when you reach this crossroad.

Marriage and Role Options

Once two people have made the decision to marry, they will enter a new stage of life with its own challenges, satisfactions and strains. An interesting way of looking at marriage has been provided by Charles Handy.[6] He has studied husbands and wives in terms of their needs for achievement, dominance, affiliation, and nurturance. As can be seen in Figure 1, he combined 'achievement' and 'dominance' needs and 'affiliation' and 'nurturance' needs, and came up with four patterns which reflect fundamental approaches to life. To arrive at particular *marriage patterns*, he combined the husbands' orientations with those of the wives.

Although there are sixteen logically possible combinations of marriage patterns, Handy's investigations turned up only eight patterns, with only four principal patterns occurring. We will look at his four most frequent ones, as shown in Figure 1. The first pattern was of a 'thrusting husband and a caring wife', which Handy found to be the most frequent pattern and the one which represents the traditional sex-role stereotype. Here the husband is the breadwinner and the wife the homemaker. His goals of success and achievement are her goals as well, and all her efforts are involved in the home and providing him with support, although

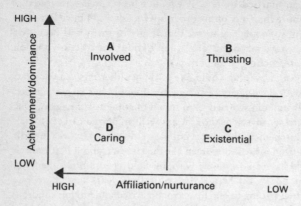

Figure 1. Types of Marriages

Source: C. Handy, 'The Family: Help or Hindrance' in C. L. Cooper and R. Payne (eds.), *Stress at Work* (Chichester. John Wiley, 1978)

she is not particularly interested in the details of his work. These marriages are predictable, structured, and create little stress. Although Handy found this marriage still to be in the majority, the prospects for its future survival are bleak.

The negative aspects of this pattern are that the wife has difficulty in expressing or meeting her own needs while her children are around. She also may find it difficult to cope when the children leave home or the husband's career reaches its ceiling, or indeed, deteriorates.

The second marriage pattern is 'the pairing of two thrusters'. In this pattern, both the husband and the wife have high needs for achievement and dominance. In the past, the thrusting wife tended to stay at home and either be frustrated at not achieving her own goals, or attempt to meet her achievement need in homemaking activities. Thrusters usually desire support or the 'caring' role, and if both are making this demand known, considerable discontent can result. This is also the pairing situation most likely to lead to dual-career families, confronting the changing conception of woman's role in the home. Naturally, if both thrusters become thoroughly involved in their worklife, as they are likely to do, their domestic arrangements and circumstances are likely to be very chaotic indeed. Since, by definition, thrusters – whether husband or wife – need the comforts of the home environment, the conflicts, tensions, and stress in the family will be enormous. In addition, these types of relationships become very much more strained when children arrive on the scene because the husband attempts to get his wife to play out the traditional sex-role stereotype (that is, she must give up her job), and draws on the guilt he knows his wife has buried just below the surface of her emancipation.

The third pattern is the partnership of two 'involved' people. Although the husband and wife are both high achievers, with a tendency to be dominant in their interpersonal relationships, they also place a high value on 'caring' and 'belonging'. As Handy suggests, 'they prefer to share arenas, not separate them'. The stress level in these marriages is very high, since both partners have an underlying 'thrusting' instinct, but this is tempered with a 'caring' element that encourages them to confront one another with problems. In contrast, two thrusters would avoid resolution by compromise and discussion, and would seek victory through defeat. Although in this third pattern one partner or the other may have to do something in the short run that he or she would prefer not to, there is sufficient flexibility in the marriage to provide short-term support so that he or she can end up doing what either wants to do in the longer term.

And finally, the last marriage pattern is an 'involved husband' with a 'caring wife'. Here the husband is highly achievement-orientated but also values the caring aspect of relationships. The husband is likely to be under a great deal of stress, since not only is he ambitious, but he also cares about other people and is very concerned not to hurt others. Because the husband is sensitive to other people's feelings, he feels guilty when his wife commits herself solely to him (although he does want her social support). As Handy suggests, these relationships are 'less predictable and the tensions less well contained. These relationships are more intense and emotional. There is more questioning and more effort to rework roles than in the traditional marriages.'

Handy makes the following points in respect of this framework and its effect on family stress:

1 Where the activity pattern of a marriage fits that which would normally be required by the underlying mix of personalities there will be less 'familial stress'. For example, if an A–A couple [see Figure 1] were forced by the success of the husband and the needs of the children to adopt a B–D pattern, family stress is likely to be increased.

2 If the pattern of husband-wife relationship didn't change with changes in the central life interests of each member, there is liable to be more family stress.

3 If there are changes in the activity pattern at home or work which do not fit with one of the satisfactory marriage patterns above, then either the job or the attitudes or the partners must change if stress and conflict are to be avoided.

Dual-career Families

The economic pressure of inflation, and more important, the social and psychological need 'to develop one's self-identity' are encouraging women to take a more active role outside the home, to pursue full-time careers or education, and to participate more widely in society generally. Indeed, Tim and Francine Hall suggest that the 'traditional family model of the husband as breadwinner and wife as homemaker, together "till death do us part", is becoming a vestige of a past society'.[7] According to the US Labor Department, the traditional 'typical American family' with a working husband, a homemaker wife, and two children, now makes up only 7 per cent of the nation's families. In addition, in 1975 44 per cent of all married women were working, as were 37 per cent of women with children under six; in 1960, the comparable figures were 31 per cent and 19 per cent, respectively.

In Britain the trend is the same. The UK male labour force has increased by 3 per cent in the last 20 years, whereas the number of women employed has grown by 43 per cent during the same period. In addition, 25 years ago there were 2.7 million married women in jobs, but by 1976 that figure rose by 142 per cent to 6.7 million. At the start of that period only a quarter of all women who were working were married; by 1976 two thirds of all working women were married. And in most European countries, the proportion of married women, with and without children, who were in full-time employment was very high (e.g., Hungary 85 per cent, Sweden 60 per cent).

It is this employment of married women more than any other development which many sociologists and psychologists are claiming is responsible for the doubling of the divorce rate over the last ten years in the US and many other countries in the West. Indeed, a review of thirteen major studies of marital adjustment in dual-career marriages showed that at least eleven studies concluded that marital adjustment was worse for dual-career wives than for non-working wives. That is not to say that this development is an unworthy one, but rather to acknowledge the reality that social change of this sort, in the short term, has led to a great deal of stress within the family, and ultimately in the individual's worklife. The problem stems primarily from the fact that the family as a social support system has declined; the family once provided the breadwinning husband with a 'safe haven' from the pressures of everyday working life – or at least that is what he had come to expect. Jean Renshaw puts this current dilemma succinctly: 'according to traditional corporate mythology, the ideal family is a support system to help each employee carry out company policy. Each morning the executive emerges from his domestic cocoon, refreshed and ready to do battle in the business world. In the evening, he returns to the family haven for solace, support, and refurbishment. If this was ever the reality, it is no longer; and the illusion is becoming increasingly difficult to maintain.'[8] She goes on to liken this traditional conception of the family to a missile system, with the company as the command module and the family as the support system. In this system, she suggests, 'message direction is fixed: control messages travel down; support and nourishment messages travel up. Inputs come from the environment of the corporation, not from feedback or give and take. The command module has the important information and "knows best".' But, as we all know, the worlds of work and home are interdependent; one set of decisions reached at work may very easily affect the home environment, and, likewise, changes in the marital situation are also likely to affect the work environment.

Because the dual-career marriage is slowly, but surely, becoming a part of Western life, it is worth noting the consequences it is likely to have on the marital relationship, the children, society and business. The viewpoints regarding this are mixed. Back in the early fifties, T. Parsons prophesied the self-destructive nature of dual-career marriages and stated that marriage between professionals was 'not a workable way of emancipating most American married women from domesticity'.[9] He based this on the socio-cultural reasons that this type of marriage could throw the wife into a destructive role competition with her husband. Indeed, high stress levels are experienced by many dual-career families. R. Pahl suggested that there is an 'infection exhaustion' caused by the strain and bustle dual-career couples are subject to.[10] The stress that is internal to the partnership derives primarily from role conflict, since dual-career couples must function satisfactorily in three roles simultaneously: marriage, child-rearing and work. 'Identity' crises are caused because of the difficulties of overcoming the societal norms of housework and family rearing being female concerns, and 'work' essentially male. Dilemmas generated by the changing of roles arise from problems encountered at the workplace at crucial stages. This stress, which comes about at job transition points, results in dual-career couples trying to avoid having more than one of the three areas of engagement (the roles outlined above) in transition at the same time. Stress might also result when one partner's career conflicts with the other's, such as a promotion for one spouse which involves a job relocation and career break for the partner.[11]

The dual-career couple's social life tends to be restricted, since they have to cope jointly with both the responsibilities of work and home. This results in their rationing out their social life and modifying their choice of friends. In the case of relatives, however, the choice cannot be made that easily and this causes many dilemmas socially, particularly for the wife, since the dual-career husband is frequently close to his mother and might find it difficult to ration his visits to her.[12]

Working wives have widely varying attitudes towards their jobs. For some women, their own jobs soon take second place to husbands and homes; they value their jobs mainly as a way of accumulating capital and because they will be able to 'take it up' again after accomplishing the immediate aim of raising a family.

This reduced involvement is often seen in a decision to change to part-time working or a willingness to take up a lower level, less time-consuming job following a geographic move. This woman has chosen to adopt a supportive role in relation to her husband's work and will make sacrifices in order to help him further his career.

At the other extreme, we have the true dual-career orientation: both partners are heavily involved in their jobs and the wife continues working because it is important to her to do so. If asked, she would undoubtedly say that she was, say, a teacher rather than subscribe to a derived identity from her role as wife. Their homebuilding is not so much 'nest preparation' as the organization of a base of operations for separate careers and joint social activities. The success of this type of relationship will depend on two basic issues: the first involves the relative importance the woman attaches to her job, her husband's job and home maintenance; the second issue centres on what expectations the husband has of the role of a wife. A consistent complaint of husbands whose wives work is that their wives become 'too involved' in the jobs they do. The working woman is in a position of obvious role conflict, especially if her job makes demands on her after 5.00 p.m., and interferes temporarily with her role as housekeeper and companion. The increasing number of women attending university has made this more likely; no longer are they necessarily secretaries and the like, with limited hours and responsibilities. Their career opportunities may now extend to the law, computer programming, management, health care, engineering, just like their husbands, and the norms and expectations in these occupations are the same as those for men. 'Equal opportunities' are generally only open to women who show themselves willing to subscribe to these norms.

The repercussions in the above marriage will depend largely on the husband's attitude and behaviour. We believe that a relatively 'New Man' is necessary to understand and accommodate a 'New Woman's' ambitions. This New Man must be willing to sacrifice home comforts (the 'home' he has come to expect from parental patterns), share the burden of maintaining the home and, most important, be able to cope with a wife who may well be successful in a world which bears comparison to his. While the roles, for example, of traditional man and wife/mother can be complementary (and enhance each other if they are both performed well), the roles of, say, male executive and female advertising agency executive can be competitive (either by salary or status differentials), and it is not easy for one to do well without being a potential threat to the other.

Many men now subscribe to the New Man ethic and take pleasure in the achievements of their partners: the behaviour of most, however, shows signs of an underlying *ambivalence*. A few covertly reinforce the values of good cooking and housekeeping, while openly denying the importance of such things, and most are happy to be fussed over (in moderation), but openly affirm the 'egalitarian mate' ideal. R. D. Laing, among other British psychiatrists, has put forward strong evidence that the reception of conflicting messages from highly valued and inescapable sources plays a part in the etiology of mental ill health. Perhaps this explains the confusion about life goals of many of today's young women.

Whatever his success in coping with these interpersonal issues at home, the working professional husband in this situation is less likely to be able to devote as much of himself to his work as did members of the previous generation. If he is a true New Man he will, by definition, value and spend time on his share of the household duties; the couple will probably also develop a pattern of sharing each other's work stresses and satisfactions as part of their emphasis on a joint lifestyle. If he is an Ambivalent New Man he is likely to find the role negotiations required to maintain his marriage both energy consuming and distracting. Both alternatives are far from the previous pattern, in which the husband was released from duties and buffered from pressure so that he could get on with his career. The egalitarian nature of the relations in this type of marriage dictates that decisions should be made jointly and with the aim of maximizing the satisfaction of both partners. This causes particularly acute problems when the couple is faced with demands from his workplace (and in the future, hers as well), such as the offer of a geographic move or a period of foreign travel. No longer can the husband accept and then go home and tell his wife. Many organizations have not yet appreciated the ramifications of this development and still negotiate doggedly with only one member of the decision-making unit. This immediately puts the employee in conflict with the couple and will add to any strain he or she already feels at not being independent.

A woman who is married to an Ambivalent New Man will eventually find she carries many of the homemaking burdens; she will rush from work to the store, and from store to home to make dinner. Unless she has help, she spends her free time on household tasks. She has less energy to put into her work and as a result may begin to despise both her husband and the organization for the pressure they are putting on her.

Once the young couple have come to terms with, or are coping fairly well with, the stress of a dual-career marriage, their next concern is whether they should have children. This question often falls back into the lap of the woman: is she to give up work and devote herself to the family, permanently or for a period, or does she find someone to look after her children while she goes to work? These choices are intrinsically stressful. The first can cause frustration and trapped feelings; the second can result in the guilt and pain of leaving the children in someone else's care. The decisions that each dual-career couple makes when considering a family will depend largely on the way their relationship has evolved and the roles each partner fills.

An interesting categorization of dual-career marriages has been designed by Francine and Tim Hall in their excellent book *The Two career Couple*.[13] Incidentally, they define the two-career couple as 'two people who share a lifestyle that includes (1) cohabitation, (2) separate work roles for both partners, and (3) a love relationship that supports and facilitates both'. They contend that there are four dual-career family role structures: accommodators, adversaries, allies, and acrobats. The *accommodator* pattern usually has one partner who is high in career involvement and low in home involvement, while the other partner is high in home involvement and low in career involvement. The difference between this pattern and the traditional family one is that either sex can play either role. The possible stresses and strains are kept to a minimum. There are an increasing number of men prepared to play the traditional female role while wives become the bread-winners – although the movement in this direction is insignificant in comparison to the number of families with working husbands and wives.

The *adversaries*, on the other hand, are very much the two working thrusters described earlier, a couple in which 'both partners are highly involved in their careers, and have low involvement in home, family, or partner support roles'. As in the two thruster marriages, this is the most stressful marital pattern, where there is competition over priorities, avoidance of non-work roles in the family, conflict in terms of career development of either member, and the unwillingness to give up any of their career identity to meet the needs of husband/wife or the family unit (unless the work costs are negligible).

The third type is the *allies* pattern in which 'two people are both highly involved in either career or home and family roles, with little identity tied up in the other'. This is broken down into two different orientations. In the former, neither partner identifies with a career. Both derive their primary satisfaction from their family and their relationship. In the other, they identify strongly with their jobs and not the family, and 'their identities are not tied up in having a well-ordered home, gourmet dinners, entertaining, or often, children. The support structure may be "purchased", in dinners out, maids, and catering services, or simply not exist.' The potential stress problem in the latter case is that the couple doesn't have the time required to maintain the relationship as a support base for their independent activities.

The fourth type of couple is the *acrobats*. As the name implies this type of couple is made up of partners who are highly involved in all their roles, both work and family. They perceive the home and work roles as equally important and, therefore, are very vulnerable to overload. As Hall and Hall suggest, their major source of stress derives from the 'conflict of trying to meet all the demands – having a successful career, being a good partner, having a well ordered home, providing real and emotional support for the spouse, and still finding time for the relationship'.

FAMILY LIFE CYCLES

The above discussion of dual-career marriages pointed out a

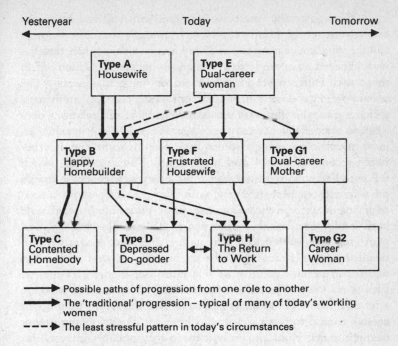

Figure 2. Profiles of Wives

Source: C. L. Cooper and J. Marshall, *Management International Review*, 1977

number of sources of stress confronting married couples today. We will now follow the family life cycle, examining the early marriage, child-rearing and 'empty nest' stages, and look more closely at the options available to women. We will also discuss the possible advantages of dual-career families.

Figure 2 shows a variety of roles played by women in Western society at different stages of the family life cycle. We are talking here primarily of white-collar employees, because they seem to be the ones experiencing the greatest stress (due to the increased mobility of the professional women). This is not to indicate that problems don't exist for blue-collar women but, because they have been in the work-force longer, these problems are less dramatic and destructive.

This look at wives' roles is organized along two axes: the first represents the family life cycle from early marriage through childbearing and rearing to the empty nest (which includes families with children at home who are relatively independent, as well as those with children who are married or living separately). The second axis is a time continuum from 'yesteryear' to 'tomorrow' which is meant to illustrate the developments in role relations over a period of time. Over twenty years ago, in many Western countries, most middle-class young women took on jobs to fill the time between secondary school and married life. Those 'careers' which followed had no long-term expectations; they were basically service posts (nurse, teacher, secretary) with poor promotional prospects, requiring no excessive involvement out of work hours, as did male jobs, and were suitable forerunners to raising children and managing the problems of a home and husband. It was typical, therefore, for a woman to give up her job as soon as she got married to become a full-time housewife (see Figure 2, Type A). This is no longer the case. Most women now continue working after marriage and add their income to their husband's to build up enough capital to 'start a home'. They usually wait longer before having the first child and only then do they possibly leave work. This 'generation gap' differentiation is depicted by Types A and E, respectively, in Figure 2. In addition, this time axis not only reflects the changing role of women, but also that of different generations and socio-economic status. Roles associated with Types A and D are or have been filled by the wives of today's more senior professional workers – those in the fifty- to sixty-five-year-old age group: all other Types are possible descriptions of the wives of the next generation of white-collar workers (although only a small number now fit the Type A characterization). The thin arrow lines on the diagram indicate possible paths of progression from one role to another. Some of the many variables which affect this progression are dealt with more fully below. The thick lines show the accepted traditional pattern, and the broken lines the least stressful pattern in today's changed conditions.

Each of these roles has a consequence for the well-being of family and home life, and for the stress levels of both the man, the woman and the children in the family.

Organizational Demands on Employees and Their Families

Before going on to look at family life in more detail, it should be pointed out that what most organizations demand and expect of their white-collar employees in return for success and promotion has not dramatically changed over the last thirty years. (It must be noted that here we assume professionals view their jobs as major sources of life satisfaction and are sufficiently ambitious to follow a developing, expanding and fulfilling career throughout their working lives. We are, therefore, concentrating on the employee who wants to get on.) Organizations expect their white-collar employees to become highly involved in the success of the company and of their own jobs in particular. They are expected to display their involvement and dedication by heavy investments of emotional energy and time, working in the evenings and at weekends when necessary, travelling on company business, spending 'appropriate' time on work-related social activities and responding enthusiastically to company offers of promotion or geographic mobility. Any free time they do have should be spent in rest and recuperation, to enable them to come back refreshed and ready for further company service.

The job demands that blue-collar workers feel may not invade so much into their home time, but can often be more physically stressful. For instance, overtime has to be taken to show commitment and to enhance the take-home pay. The blue-collar worker, therefore, will come home physically and often mentally tired (he or she, too, experiences the work stress factors mentioned in Chapter 4) and, just like the white-collar worker, his or her free time is still seen by the company as a means by which the worker can recuperate. By no means should home problems interfere with work.

Taking these work demands into account, and putting the alternative roles of both husband and wife back into the context of the marriage, we can now see what the implications of the individual choices are when establishing families.

Child-rearing Phase

At this phase of family life, the economic burden of the blue-collar working family does not offer choices; women must and often do work. They may enjoy that work or may wish they could provide more of the caring roles of a woman at home. The stresses and strains of family and home life tend to be those of financial difficulties, coping with the demands of home and children (often the blue-collar male is more reluctant to take on the traditional female caretaking roles) and providing a comfortable home base for all the family. Blue-collar, like white-collar, working women have the same problems of finding good child caretaking facilities and coping when a child is ill and off from school. They must decide who goes to the school to meet teachers or see a child perform in school activities. These demands all cause strains in marriages and in relationships with children, particularly for certain family structures.

Happy Homebuilder and Traditional Man

Most white-collar and middle-class women, however, have a number of alternatives as seen in Figure 2. This has implications for the well-being of the woman, her husband and their children.

One alternative is the 'happy homebuilder'. This woman is, in most cases, the housewife who subjugates her career to her husband's and begins a family. The phase of happy homebuilder is an extremely important one for a woman, especially for those with no career ambitions. It is a time for exploring and establishing an extremely fulfilling, but demanding and time-consuming role. The young wife's preoccupation now parallels her husband's involvement in his job. This phase is one of relatively few problems. The couple's relationship is, however, likely to be somewhat distanced and their roles highly differentiated, and for many this will mean they don't 'meet' psychologically very often. As with the other facets of their lives, the couple are likely to keep many of their problems separate. Because he wants to preserve a 'safe haven' in which to shut out work matters, and because much of his job will be too confidential and technical for 'her to understand', the man tends not to bring his work stresses home to his wife. She, in turn, will keep many of her own problems to herself, in order to protect him from extra strain, to avoid negative feedback, to preserve his image of her as a loving and supportive wife, and in addition, because their real time together is too precious to waste.

She may also buffer him from the demands of the children ('Daddy's tired, leave him alone now') and the organizational aspects of running a home (such as house moving, arranging holidays, organizing house repairs). By protecting each other in this way, the working husband and his wife are also shielding themselves from having to share and handle the stresses of the other. They are deeply involved in deriving satisfaction from their separate worlds, and their shared pleasures are mainly when they 'meet' through their children. The husband is free to devote himself to work, and his wife's activities directly support him in this by providing a stable, comfortable home, a ready-made and undemanding low-stress identity system (husband and father) and, in addition, local social contacts (often, again, via the children). This is a life of 'complementary' rather than 'shared' relationships.

Frustrated Housewife, Traditional Man

While many women solve their problem by acknowledging a 'need' to bear and raise children and, therefore, drop out of their careers to become 'happy homebuilders' (usually planning to return to work later), some take on the role of mother only to deeply regret their action later. It is such women who are potential 'frustrated housewives'; they are not happy with the role of mother and housekeeper in which they find themselves. It is not generally that these women have been tricked into motherhood by unwanted pregnancy – they have usually decided to have children because they felt that they might find it satisfying or that they might later regret not having done so, or in response to social pressure from parents, friends, or husbands. Once there, they are trapped. Generally, however, they are well-educated enough to know about the effects of parental neglect on young children and set high standards for their mothering role; few would even consider working before their children are five years old and many feel that they should wait until their children are of secondary school age (twelve years old). Even if they would like to work, many have careers which cannot be pursued part-time or which necessitate living near a major city. Not only do these women derive little intrinsic enjoyment from the day-to-day activities of running a home and raising a family, but they feel that they are actually suffering from the experience. Without the intellectual and social stimulations of the jobs they know they are capable of and happy doing, they feel that they are in danger of becoming 'vegetables'. The task of bringing up children, by its very nature, is a constant battle against overwhelming odds, and most mothers feel that they perform badly – for the thwarted career woman, particularly, being a mother may not be an adequately meaningful identity.

There is little positive action the frustrated housewife can take, and usually she directs her negative feelings at the nearest target – her husband. He has everything she lacks and also reaps the benefits of her grudging labours. She is jealous of his work and any time he devotes to it (she may well resent him working late or socializing after work, for example); she will discourage him from bringing work home, either physically or psychologically (as a problem or a triumph), and she certainly will be loath to play the 'social, dutiful wife' role, which in some organizations is essential to his career progress.

The husband facing this type of home situation often feels that he, too, is trapped. However sympathetic he may be, and as much as he tries to supply continuous support, there are no easy practical solutions to his wife's problems. The strain this imposes on him, at what might well be a crucial time in his career, is considerable, and may seriously affect his work performance. Problems with relationships at home are likely to affect work in the following ways: (a) releasing tensions into relationships at work; (b) cramming work into a nine-to-five day to avoid bringing work home, creating work overload; (c) basing career decision-making partly on his wife's hostility towards his work (for example, refusing greater responsibilities or travel commitments). It would not be surprising in the admittedly extreme situation we have depicted for the husband to partly lose patience with his wife's frustrations and send her 'stress messages' in turn: 'Life would be a lot simpler if I didn't have a wife and family'; 'You were a much nicer person to know when you were out at work'; 'It's not surprising that I prefer to spend time at work rather than listening to your moaning.'

The passage of time, rather than 'active coping', provides the usual solution to problems of couples in this role tangle. The husband misses career advancement opportunities and compensates by reducing his ambitions and putting his family first in importance; as children grow up the wife becomes freer to look outside the home for meaningful activities. But there are signs that changes in society are helping to alleviate some of the problems: flexitime allows many employees to tailor their work hours to fit home demands; some firms are encouraging job sharing (two part-time people sharing one job), which allows women to be involved in work and child care; and career-break schemes initiated by the banks help career women during early child-rearing. Local community groups belonging to the National Housewives' Register organize activities for young mothers who prefer not to talk about the problems of washing nappies; 'babysitting circles' free couples from the home more regularly; and local colleges offer interesting and mind-developing courses in everything from pottery to the degree subjects that will help in the resumption of (paid) work in later life.

Dual-career Mother

The measures mentioned at the end of the previous section are all aimed at making the sacrifices a career woman undertakes in the child-rearing phase more palatable. An alternative, however, is to obviate the need for such sacrifice altogether, by following a continuous dual-career progression – with short interruptions for childbearing. Here we see many of the problems discussed above for the newly married dual-career couple, but with some added complications. Firstly, child-rearing (unlike dish-washing) cannot be neglected without serious repercussions. To date, there have been few comprehensive and readily available child-care facilities in many countries. Secondly, the woman's decision to continue, rather than break and resume, her work means that she is as able to develop a career successfully as her husband. This fact intensifies her problem of managing time and involvement with regard to work, and may increase her husband's susceptibility to feeling threatened by her competition. Thirdly, compared to the household of the 'frustrated housewife', in which the norm is that the husband's job should be denied importance (with under-achievement a consequence), the husband of a career woman is likely to be expected to place high emphasis on his work, devote time to it, and succeed. In this situation, the husband could well push himself more at work, courting the strain of overpromotion. Unlike the husband of the happy homebuilder, the career woman's husband will lack the back-up of the supportive wife with plenty of time to help him cope with work stresses (she may well have plenty of her own), and a ready-made social world in which he can unwind. It may also become important not to be left behind if his wife is successful. Fourthly, shortage of time and preoccupation with work may well mean that the couple adopts a slightly distant relationship similar to that seen in the happy homebuilder, but without the tacitly agreed priorities of the latter; decision-making in the dual-career family could, therefore, be a traumatically divisive activity. Personality characteristics will play a large part in the success of this type of marriage – the benefits of a family pattern which simultaneously satisfies the needs of all its members are obvious. If, however, the couple are both achievement-orientated and conscientious, they may well take on more than they can jointly manage.

The strains of a dual-career family on both the husband and wife can be great, the burdens of which (finding adequate childminders; handling the management of a home; successfully filling the expectations that children at school have of parents; dealing with illness and sudden family crises) can all become an excessive burden. This, along with work stress and feelings of guilt at not being able to cope with either world successfully, can cause a major breakdown either emotionally or physically. The woman may experience this type of stress more if her partner is the Ambivalent New Man or, indeed, the Traditional Man because these men are less likely to share the household management tasks. The Ambivalent Man may want to, but is unable mentally to adapt to domestic situations and problems, having probably grown up in a traditional family situation with a happy homebuilder mother.

Favourable Consequences of a Dual Career

Instead of destroying the institution of marriage, dual-career families may well cause a strengthening of marital ties.[14] The increase in the employment of wives brings about a more symmetrical family structure in which a greater degree of equality can prevail between husband and wife.[15] When the wife works, the couple's resources tend to be equalized which, in turn, affects the power structure of the family. We see a 'companionship family' developing, in which the husband pays more attention to what his wife says, and she begins to treat him as an equal instead of 'putting him on a pedestal'. The effect of this is that her powers grow (relatively), while his decline. This companionship family may well be a new stage in the history of the family in the West.[16] These dual-career couples act more jointly in directing their internal responsibilities and tend to choose their friends more jointly than the traditional couple. Even in a pessimistic Ohio study, confidence was felt in the ties of mutual trust which develop in the marital relationship where both husband and wife participate increasingly in the decision-making.[17]

For children, too, there are favourable consequences of a dual-career family. The working mother will influence her children, but not in the way suggested by the commonly held prejudice – namely, that mothers who are not in constant attendance on their children risk nurturing delinquents. The same sort of role convergence that takes place between husband and wife can also be seen between son and daughter. Daughters of working mothers are more self-sufficient, independent and disobedient. Seeing their mother work, according to researchers, encourages daughters to take up part-time and summer employment.[18] They do this while, at the same time, increasing their share of the housework. Seeing the females in their family becoming equal with them, however, somehow has the effect of demoralizing sons in the short term. This might be explained by the fact that they are modelling themselves on their fathers, who are no longer feeling responsible for providing monetary support for the family. The boys tend to become more meek and obedient, as Hoffman suggests, reflecting the lower status of their fathers.[19] In other words, the boys become less masculine and the girls become more masculine, neither of which is an undesirable trend, but merely brings about role convergence and increased equality among sexes.

Advantages have been found to accrue to children when the mothers works. Working women are less demanding of their children, since they have devoted less time and effort in bringing them up. Moreover, children no longer have to feel guilty about their

Table 1. The Advantages and Disadvantages of Marriage Orientations

	Men		Women
	Advantages	Disadvantages	Advantages
Happy homemaker. Traditional Man	He will be able to pursue a career without hindrance and have a place to recuperate.	He is unable to share his work problems, can feel alienated from his wife. Sees family little.	Happy building home, looking after the children.
Frustrated wife. Traditional Man	Has a home base where he may find respite.	Home is not calm, may have to listen to wife's problems. She is not interested in his problems, wife demands more of his time. He has no excuse in the eyes of his company.	None: believes she is doing what is right, looking after the children.
Career mother. Ambivalent New Man	Feels he is modern, doing what his counterparts are doing.	Still wants the comforts. Wants to spend time at work – has to share responsibilities. Feels he is not able to put all his effort into his job, therefore detrimental to his career. May feel in competition with his wife.	Enjoys continuing career, feels fulfilled intellectually.
Career mother. New Man	Enjoys having an egalitarian marriage. Strengthened marital ties.	Lacks the back-up of a wife at home and a ready-made social world to relax in. May take on too much, both at home and at work. May find his career adversely affected.	Enjoys continuing career, feels fulfilled. Has the support of her husband.

Children

Disadvantages	Advantages	Disadvantages
Has little in common with husband, may have to deal with home problems alone.	A secure and stable home life with mother.	May have very little contact with father.
Jealous of husband, feels she will become a vegetable, feels frustrated and under-used – has no self-respect.	Mother is at home to provide all needs.	Parents in conflict, mother frustrated. She may take it out on them.
Feels the burden of home tasks as husband is not pulling his weight. Worries about leaving the children. Has to deal predominantly with child-care problems. Coping with three roles at once.	Both parents are stimulated. Mother happy.	Less ease and comfort at home. May feel rejected. Parents in debate as to roles and responsibilities.
Still has to deal with domestic problems – jointly with her husband. The home and work demands may cause undue strain. Her career may be adversely affected.	Children may be more self-sufficient and independent. Have modern role models for both sexes.	Less ease and comfort at home. Children can be more independent but also more disobedient.

mothers sacrificing their careers for them.[20] The attitudes among children towards female employment become more positive when their mothers work. A study of 1,055 ninth-grade children in the United States revealed that those whose mothers worked looked upon this employment as less of a threat to the marriage relationship than did children of non-working mothers.[21] This effect was found to be more significant for males than for females. To sum up, we can say that the employment of the mother leads to a convergence of roles of the husband and wife, and of son and daughter, whereby they all participate more in common activities and share in closer family life.

There are advantages and disadvantages of all the marriage orientations illustrated in Table 1. But it is critical for the well-being of the family as a whole that the partners in a marriage identify what their needs are, and try to accommodate them. These accommodations can involve trying to find satisfying part-time work for the frustrated housewife (even if the money she earns goes in paying for child-minders) or getting more domestic help for the dual-career couple.

Empty Nest Phase

The phase in which children become more independent and, indeed, leave home, often has a new set of stress factors and strains for husband and wife – most of which are related to the previous child-rearing phase. For instance, if the wife is willing to continue to maintain a supportive role *vis-à-vis* her husband, we would describe her as a 'contented homebody'. As her family duties decrease, she may well take on outside activities such as volunteer work, tennis, or painting, to fill the time once occupied by children. If her husband has done well in his career she may well take on a social role in relation to his job by entertaining visitors, acting as a resource for his subordinates' wives, or providing a social focus for his department. If she adopts the latter type of role, she is likely to derive much of her social identity from her husband's status. In this kind of marriage, where the couple continue in their complementary roles, the husband is often extremely successful at work; many would say that the organization has benefited by getting one and a half employees for the price of one.

Behaviourally it is not easy to distinguish the contented homebody from the potential role we have labelled 'depressed do-gooder'. But while they may fill their days in the same way, the latter does not find the things she does fulfilling. Often she will pick up and drop a series of hobbies and local community activities, looking for one to give her life 'meaning' – but without success. Usually, too, she is prevented from getting a 'proper' job as a possible outlet because she has no marketable job skills or lacks the confidence and training opportunities to resurrect any she did have, and also because both she and her husband have been brought up to believe that he should support her.

How then, do the contented homebodies and the depressed do-gooders come to differ so radically in their outlook on life? Consistently we find that while the former has built up a meaningful identity, the latter has failed to do so. There could be various reasons for this – perhaps geographic moves or upward social mobility has disrupted her life and prevented her from becoming integrated into a stimulating society, or perhaps she has not been able to derive meaning from her husband's work. Whatever the reasons, the wife in these circumstances is likely to be unhappy and frequently depressed. Though she may turn to her husband for support, he may well be in no position to help her – if his job is still demanding, he will not have the time or energy to spare for his wife's rather vague identity problems; it may be that he also shows signs of stress (perhaps because he has reached his career ceiling) and is facing the problem of lack of meaning in his life too. Such a couple are likely to find these circumstances extremely stressful, particularly if they developed a rather distanced relationship in their earlier married life; they are now hampered by their lack of experience in dealing with interpersonal problems of this nature.

Re-entering the World of Work

During the empty nest phase, some women return to work. This re-entry could be at a time when the wife feels her family is sufficiently able to cope with such a development, and may well be part-time at first, to fit in with their demands. Trends towards smaller families (to release women from family demands earlier), and the fact that many middle-aged women are robbed of most of the grandparenting duties because their offspring are highly mobile, have helped to make an early return to work increasingly more likely. Other motivating reasons may be the desire to supplement the family income, a need for achievement and satisfaction, or an attempt to maintain a separate life to compensate for a husband too dedicated to his work.

The family implications of 'the return' depend largely on which type of relationship the couple have progressed from. The happy homebody and traditional husband may initially have difficulty because she was not sufficiently interested in education when younger to acquire marketable skills. If, however, she can overcome such problems, both she and her husband are likely to benefit. Typically, she will guard against her job intruding in any way on the supportive pattern she and her husband have built up; as long as she maintains his job as their primary consideration, he can only gain from her added interest in life. One husband remarked, in a recent study, how pleased he was to see his wife enjoying her job so much, 'She re-became the woman I married.' This 'new wife' may later play an important part as a sharer of activities, as her husband nears retirement and his job demands less of his energies.

For the woman who does not limit her new work activities to fit in with home demands, the situation is likely to be more difficult, especially if her husband has come to expect a particularly high level of home comfort. Conscientious dual-career families will have negotiated issues earlier; previous happy homebuilders are likely to experience some initial friction, but as we said earlier, the husband's needs usually take priority in any situation of conflict such as this. It is the frustrated housewife who is likely to be the most excessive in her demands for work satisfaction. The couple for whom this is true are likely to undergo yet another period of turmoil, as they attempt to establish a new balance in their relationship. The husband now has some hope of favourable outcomes and looks forward to the release of previous tensions. His wife, however, is likely to be under considerable strain as she re-enters the world of work, of which she has high expectations of satisfaction – which may not be fully met by the local labour market. Provided that these issues can be successfully worked out, the wife's return to work is likely to be beneficial to both partners.

The career woman who has maintained her career throughout child-rearing, should not have the problems of transition back to work, during the empty nest phase. It should be a good opportunity for getting ahead in her career. If, however, she has major career ambitions at an age incompatible with those ambitions and the job's requirements, she may become frustrated. Her husband, as already discussed, may reach a career ceiling and may want to wind down towards retirement, hoping to spend more time with his wife and not be in career competition. This can create conflict.

The empty nest years for a man, therefore, can either be years of relative peace and contentment or another upheaval, not only at home but in his job (as discussed in Chapter 4). He may have achieved success, be burnt out or on the edge of retirement, and he will perceive more or less stress depending on his home-life situation and his social support.

The stresses of the empty nest years, as any other phase, are clearly dependent on the individual characteristics of the family, its financial and geographic location and many complex factors. In highlighting the alternative roles, as we have done, we can identify where potential problems may and do arise. For instance, the 'happy homemaker', 'contented homebody', and 'the traditional man' may have successfully completed their early child-rearing years by keeping their family and working lives relatively separate, as part of different worlds; when thrown together in the empty nest years or in retirement they may find they have nothing in common. The 'frustrated wife' during this phase may have found an outlet for her frustration, and may be more content with herself and her husband. He may feel released of the burden of a wife and family, can enjoy his later years of work and savour them with his re-invigorated, 'liberated wife'.

Who Wins?

Figure 3 suggests a 'Who Wins' table for three of the actors in the field of home and work – the husband, wife and husband's or wife's employing organization. 'Winning' essentially means matching expectations and needs, whatever these may be, with reality.

We see that while the traditional marriage progression (A–B–C) might lack some of the personal contact and growth elements advocated today, overall it was beneficial to the husband, and to his firm, and it assigned a stable role to the wife (if a limiting one). In it, relationships struck some kind of balance. The marriage patterns

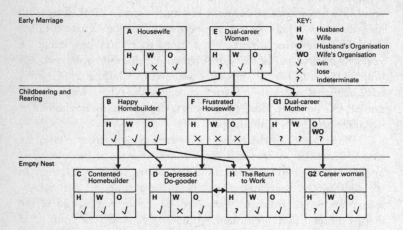

Figure 3. 'Who Wins' Table: Wives' Roles and Win/Lose Consequences for the Husband, Wife, and Organizations

Source: C. L. Cooper and J. Marshall, *Management International Review*, 1977.

of today contain new conflicts and ambiguities, which mean that equilibrium must be established individually by negotiation, rather than taken for granted. While the bonds arrived at between husband and wife have the potential to be exceedingly rich and rewarding, their establishment and maintenance does require an expenditure of energy on the husband's part not previously demanded. In many cases his, or her, organizations will find people less able and probably less willing to devote themselves wholeheartedly to its goals in the short term. In the long term, however, organizations may reap the benefits of more harmonious family relationships.

RECURRENT ISSUES AND HOME-LIFE STRESS

We have looked at alternative family structures and the implications these alternatives have for the individual, the family and the employer in turn. Within all of these structures, there will be recurrent events and issues which can add to 'life stress'.[22]

Life Events

As discussed in Chapter 3, life events can have a powerful effect on one's stress equilibrium. A death or divorce can seriously disrupt a person's outlook, relationships and health. It can increase stress levels enormously, and the ramifications can be felt in the home and work environment for a long time. What may be considered more minor events, such as an illness of a friend, will also have ramifications, although they may be indirect. For example, an increase in job responsibility through promotion may adversely affect the quality of time spent with family.

Divorce and Single Parenthood

One of the most stressful life events is divorce, and its primary consequence, single parenthood. The figures for divorce in most Western countries are still on the increase and growing (in England and Wales from 2 per 1000 existing marriages in 1960 to 11 per 1000 in 1980). Most psychological studies on the impact of divorce and separation suggest that all parties concerned (husband, wife, children) experience a range of emotions, from guilt to anger to projection to feelings of loss of self-worth. People involved in this traumatic event usually go through a series of stages: shock, despair, depression, loneliness, lowered self-esteem and then recovery. Once they have recovered reasonably well, the partners still have to cope with either being the single parent or the visiting parent. Both of these roles put undue pressure on the individual, which in most cases lasts a long time, particularly as circumstances continually change (such as remarriage, relocation of one parent, and so on). An awareness of the long-term effect of the stress involved in divorce, and its inevitably unresolvable nature are important realities to keep in mind. Obviously, divorce is such a complex topic that we do not have the space available to do it justice – many books are available, however, that explore it in depth.

Relocation

It is now estimated that United Kingdom managers change jobs about once every three years. Research in North America and other Western countries suggests that managerial mobility there is increasing even more rapidly. But relocation, although more frequent among middle-class/white-collar workers, does not affect them alone. With the decline in the economy in the last ten years and the increase in blue-collar unemployment, workers in the mining and steel industries have been encouraged to 'up sticks' and leave their home town for greener pastures.

Whatever the background one comes from, moving can be a traumatic and stressful event, depending on two factors. The first involves the situation in which the individual is involved, or his or her 'life area', such as job, family, and outside activities. The second factor involves characteristics of the individual – age, qualifications, job skills, and personality, that is, the base from which he or she views and interprets the world.

A WIFE'S BURDEN DURING RELOCATION

'What is often not realized by the bank is the tremendous burden moving house places on the wife. Buying and selling houses is very time consuming, the average length of time for our moves being about six months. A promotion move occurs at any time; it may be a "difficult" time in the school year for children, the housing market may be awkward, the list is endless, but the bank takes very little account of any of the problems, and it is generally the wife who has the responsibility of sorting out the difficulties. The bank's attitude is that "wives like new carpets and curtains, therefore, they enjoy moving house!" This really annoys me – generalizing about women. Bank wives are not expected to "think", just to accept! We are supposed to conform to a set model –

that of the perfect housewife, ready to comply to the demands of a husband's career, to enjoy homemaking but not to get so attached to our homes that we object to giving them up, to be totally dependent on our husbands, both financially and emotionally, yet capable of living apart for long periods, with the added ability of being a financial and legal organizer of the complexities and difficulties which surround buying and selling homes in two different parts of the country. The stereotyped role of the bank wife is full of contradictions.

'It is not only the difficulties which surround the operation of buying and selling houses which bank wives have to cope with. The financial rewards of a promotion are negligible and often, for the first twelve months after a house move, people are financially worse off than before promotion. Also a promotion carries exactly the same salary rise whether it involves a house move or not, so you don't even have the dubious consolation of a higher income to make up for all the disruptions and upsets to family life a house move can incur.'

Cary Cooper and Judi Marshall carried out a study which explored the stresses and strains of job transfer on middle and senior executives in the United Kingdom.[23] This study can help illustrate some of the problems for the individual relocating at different stages in life.

For instance, younger men in the sample reported problems such as the pressure of starting a new job (at a critical and closely watched phase in their careers); the culture shock of starting work after life at university; having no separate world to retire to in the evenings to help switch off; the problems of house hunting; being lonely in a strange town (often peopled by 'contented' married couples); leaving friends behind and trying to maintain contacts (perhaps with a possible future wife).

For young marrieds, it appeared that most couples felt free and willing to meet the challenge of a new community; it is typically at this time that they have most friends and activities outside the home. Their lack of constraints makes it easier to follow one or the other's career, to be more mobile. In a dual-career marriage complications arise: is one partner to sacrifice his or her career for the promotional move of the other? How does the partner find another rewarding occupation after the move? If both have a busy career, how do they manage the complexities of finding a new home and moving, and are they able, in their limited spare time, to begin new social relationships?

For married couples with a young family, the problems of relocations are complex, both for the more traditional marriage, where the wife is at home, and for the dual-career family. For the latter, house hunting becomes a major problem, both because the wife is too tied down to participate much, and because house choice becomes more crucial and the criteria more exacting. Size and nearness to schools and shops become important and, for the housebound wife, potential friends must also be considered. Separation is an emotionally draining time for all the family. If the wife is at home her adaption to and happiness in her new environment become critical factors. The couple may find it harder to make out-of-work friends, tied down as they are, and place more emphasis on 'nearness' (the neighbours) and 'same-boat' acquaintances (couples with children of the same age and interests). They must find new social support systems, and new child and home help if they both work.

The children, as Ivancevich suggests, are also affected by the move:

certain age groups are more susceptible to relocation stress. Pre-schoolers experience feelings of loss and insecurity. They may even interpret a relocation as a form of punishment. A young child may revert to infantile behaviour such as thumb-sucking and bed-wetting or they may experience more nightmares. Children in grade school may experience similar feelings of insecurity. Teenagers, to whom peer approval and relationships are so important, frequently have a particularly difficult time.[24]

Relocation is, therefore, an extremely stressful event at this stage.

Empty nesters, many of whom are still moving at this stage of life, may have come to regard mobility as an acceptable way of life. Others, though, express concern that they never settle down anywhere, and that they are not providing a stable home for their children and grandchildren to visit. Choosing retirement sites becomes a problem for those who have lived in so many places and belonged to none.

Relocation is a recurring problem, often inducing stress among a number of family members. In the 1980s and 1990s, with more women pursuing careers, the prospects for professional men or women being available for rapid deployment will substantially decrease. This will create a number of stressful choices for the partners in terms of the direction and the security of his or her career.

Personal Circumstances

There are a number of events like relocation which shift our lives, but are often more intrinsic to our situation or lifestyle. We might call these 'personal circumstances' which crop up at any point in life. Many people will face money worries owing to the inflation which has beset the UK in the last few years. This problem produces worries such as how to pay a mortgage, or requires people to dig deeper into savings to keep ahead of monthly bills. These nagging sources of stress acting in combination with other work or home stress, can cause mental or physical ill health. The sudden event of losing one's job or one's breadwinner is a more catastrophic event, and this alone can be extremely dangerous to health.

Another personal circumstance can involve where we live. Some people choose to live in an urban or city environment, and although they may enjoy the rush and tumble of the lifestyle, the constant noise, polluted air and cramped environment may not help relieve stress from home or work and may be physically dangerous to one's health. Of course, the poor may have little choice but to live in urban poverty-stricken neighbourhoods and suffer stress factors common to those areas, such as poor law enforcement or bad community relations, resulting in violence, theft, and physical and residential insecurity. More affluent people who choose to live outside a city, but have jobs within it, have the stress of travelling to and from work, which means they do not spend as much time with other members of the family.

Associated with the choice of residence and place of work

can come the stress of belonging to a minority group, as we have discussed in Chapter 4. In addition to that found in the workplace, ethnic minorities often encounter stress from living in a mixed community. Indeed, Ivancevich suggests that 'race and class are sociopsychological sources of stress; for example, insecurity is more likely to be found in low economic class black persons because the survival struggle taxes them physically and psychologically'.[25] In his review of the literature on race differences, A. Pettigrew presented evidence that there was a higher rate of physical illness and shorter life expectancy among blacks.[26] Security is threatened more among blacks because of higher rates of divorce and separation, loss of employment, and by fewer opportunities to support a family. Blacks from low or middle economic classes have higher rates of premature and abnormal births than white counterparts. Research seems to indicate that blacks are exposed to a higher number of these types of stress factors than their social class counterparts among whites.

The Stress of Being Unemployed

With over three million people on the dole in Britain, the stress of being unemployed is a growing topic of concern, and a problem faced by many, from the unskilled to the professional worker. In a recent review of all the research on the psychological experience of being unemployed, D. Fryer and R. Payne suggest that there is a variety of possible negative consequences.[27] Studies indicate that unemployed workers and professionals can suffer from lower levels of personal happiness, life dissatisfaction, lowered self-esteem, lower levels of psychological well-being, increased depression, difficulty in concentrating and other minor to severe behavioural problems.

In addition, there is a growing literature which suggests a strong link between physical illness and unemployment stress. In Australia, one study found that the unemployed, in contrast to the employed, reported significantly more symptoms of bronchitis, ear, nose and throat problems, as well as allergies. In a similar British study, similar results were found, with the added complications of obstructive lung disease and coronary heart disease.

Although there is a difference of opinion about the relationship of unemployment and mortality, evidence is emerging of a positive association, with studies indicating that long-term unemployment may adversely affect the longevity of the unemployed by as many as two to three years, depending on when the person had been made redundant.

All in all, the experience of being unemployed in terms of your social identity, family roles and the whole range of relationships with others is a heavy burden, the costs to society of which are enormous and to the individual incalculable. Many books are available for those who want to go into greater detail.[28]

CONCLUSION

Home-life stress is dependent upon an extremely complicated series of factors, some of which are illustrated in Table 2. Although little research has been carried out to identify the major stress agents, it is commonly recognized that these exist and can adversely affect our mental and physical well-being. Perhaps the more we are aware of the dangers, the better able we may be to take precautions before an event. Or, if we are not able to pre-empt stress, hopefully we can take action to alleviate it.

Table 2. Summary of Life Stress at Home

The need to succeed:

constant push and drive generated by self, partner, parents, organizations towards successful career, financial and status circumstances.

Marital relationships:

conflicts of home and work life, struggling to maintain relationships amidst the changing roles of men and women.

Relationships with children:

conflicts of time spent with children, work- and home-life pressures, concern over their health and education and responsibility for their future.

Personal circumstances and life events:

the unexpected traumatic event, or constant aggravation of personal circumstances, such as divorce, single parenthood, financial insecurity, etc.

Chapter Six

COPING WITH WORK STRESS

'In order that people may be happy in their work, these three things are needed: they must be fit for it; they must not do too much of it; and they must have a sense of success in it.'   John Ruskin, 1851.

As we have seen in Chapter 4, work stress can create physical and emotional problems for people. For each individual there is a potential range of factors that will put him or her under stress. 'Stimulating pressure' will change to 'debilitating stress' when the individual feels unable to cope, becomes anxious about those 'feelings of inability' and begins to adopt defensive behaviours. Once a person experiences stress, he or she will adopt a series of behaviours in reaction to it. In most cases these reactions will deal directly with the stressful situation by producing solutions to it. Typical stress agents and adaptive behaviours might be:

Stress agent	Adaptive behaviour
Overwork	Delegates some work
Lack of awareness of a particular company policy	Finds out what policy is
Poor working relationship with colleague	Confronts issue with colleague and negotiates better relationship
Underpromotion	Leaves organization for another
Company versus family demands	Negotiates with boss more 'family time' (e.g. less travel)
Role ambiguity	Seeks clarification with colleagues or superior

Each of these behaviours takes the basic source of the stress and solves it, at least temporarily, and perhaps permanently.

An alternative set of behaviours includes those which are maladaptive in that they do not deal with the problem; they avoid the problem and probably aggravate it. Typical of these might be:

Stress agent	Maladaptive behaviour
Overwork	Accepts work overload with result that general performance deteriorates
Unawareness of a particular company policy	Guesses inappropriately
Poor working relationship with colleague	Attacks colleague indirectly through third party
Underpromotion	Loses confidence and becomes convinced of own inadequacy
Company versus family demands	Blames company for family discontent
Role ambiguity	Withdraws from some aspects of work role

In all the above situations, there is something the individual and the organization can do to transform maladaptive behaviours, which are harmful to the person and those around him or her, into adaptive behaviours. Let's first explore what the individual can do to cope with stress at work. We will then focus on what the work organization can do.

WHAT INDIVIDUALS SHOULD DO TO HELP THEMSELVES

Becoming Assertive
Many of the problems individuals face at work are linked to their own inability to be assertive in their relationships with work colleagues, bosses, and even subordinates. This can reflect itself in allowing work overload, long hours, frequent travel and a range of

inappropriate activities, which can be individually and organizationally counterproductive. The assertive person is 'open and flexible, genuinely concerned with the rights of others, yet at the same time able to establish very well his or her own rights'.[1] There are fundamental differences between assertive, non-assertive, and aggressive behaviour: when you are assertive you are acknowledging your own rights and those of others; when non-assertive you are denying your own rights; and when aggressive, denying the rights of others. Psychologist Sandra Langrish gives a good example of this:

Imagine, for example, you are working on a project. It is 4.30 p.m. and you have arranged to meet a friend at 5.00 p.m. so that you can go for a meal and a theatre visit together. Your boss rushes into your office waving a piece of paper. He has just received a telephone call about some aspect of the project which requires the preparation of an additional document, '. . . right now!' You realize it will take until at least 5.45 to do the work. What do you say?

Non-assertive Response: 'That's OK. I'll drop what I'm doing and do it right now. Just leave it with me. I'll take care of it.'

Aggressive Response: 'What do you take me for? Do you think I've got nothing better to do than jump when you whistle? Well, if you do, you've got a big shock coming! I'm going out with a friend, and I'm leaving at 5.00 on the dot. Just find someone else to run after you.'

Assertive Response: 'I realize that it's important that this is done as soon as possible but I've made arrangements to meet a friend at 5.00 p.m., so I can't do it now. However, I'll do it first thing tomorrow.'[2]

Langrish's account illustrates some of the basic individual rights which women as well as men should hope to achieve by being assertive, which are:

- the right to make mistakes
- the right to set one's own priorities
- the right for one's own needs to be considered as important as the needs of other people
- the right to refuse requests without having to feel guilty
- the right to express oneself as long as one doesn't violate the rights of others
- the right to judge one's own behaviour, thoughts and emotions, and to take responsibility for the consequences

Keeping in mind the differences between aggressiveness and assertiveness, many individuals would benefit from assertiveness training. The goal of assertiveness training is to help people to learn to solve problems and enable them to say, 'I feel OK about myself. I don't have to make others feel not OK in order for me to get my needs met. I know what I want. I feel good about myself and others. I can think and I have confidence to ask for what I want.'

Individual Assertiveness Exercises

There are a number of exercises which people can do to better understand their assertive, non-assertive and aggressive behaviour in a variety of situations. Sandra Langrish has outlined a five-stage approach to understanding and doing something about being more assertive.*

Stage 1: The Assertion Self-Assessment Table. Along the left-hand side of the grid in Table 1 (see p. 164) there are headings which list a variety of activities that represent the major categories of assertiveness: expression of positive feelings, expression of self-affirmation and expression of negative feelings. The column headings list people to whom these feelings may be addressed. The people represented do not include all the people with whom you may interact; you must choose which individuals are most relevant for you.

To assess the level of assertiveness in each activity, ask yourself, 'To what extent do I feel comfortable carrying out this activity with this person?' For example, if you begin with the upper-left-hand cell you would form the question, 'Do I feel comfortable giving compliments to my boss?' If the answer is yes, enter a tick in the cell; if the answer is no, enter a cross. Continue in this manner for all the cells of the grid. Completion of the table permits the identification of those people and activities with which you have difficulty in behaving assertively.

Stage 2: Assertive Behaviour Hierarchy. From the information gained from Table 1, it is possible to construct an Assertive Behaviour Hierarchy (Table 2). To construct the hierarchy, select as the first item, a person or activity which you feel you could handle assertively with only minimal anxiety. Continue to order the items from the least to the most

---

* We should like to thank Sandra Langrish for permission to use this material on assertiveness training, published in *Improving Interpersonal Relations* (see note 2).

Table 1. Work Assertion Self-assessment Table

ACTIVITY	PEOPLE Boss	Colleagues	Subordinates	Customers	Secretary	Work friends	Business contacts
Expressing positive feelings							
Giving compliments							
Receiving compliments							
Making requests, e.g., asking for favours, help, etc.							
Initiating and maintaining conversations							
Self-affirmation standing up for your legitimate rights							
Refusing requests							
Expressing personal opinions, including disagreement							
Expressing negative feelings							
Expressing justified annoyance and displeasure							
Expressing justified anger							

Source: adapted from M. D. Galassi and J. P. Galassi, *Assert Yourself*, (New York: Human Sciences Press, 1977)

Table 2. Your Own Assertive Behaviour Hierarchy

Instructions: To construct your own hierarchy select as the first item or situation something you feel you could handle assertively with only minimal anxiety (e.g. dealing with an annoying switchboard operator). Continue to order your items from least anxiety-provoking to most anxiety-provoking. The last items should be the behaviours or situations that cause you the greatest anxiety and discomfort.

1. _____

2. _____

3. _____

4. _____

5. _____

6. _____

7. _____

8. _____

9. _____

10. _____

Continue items if necessary.

anxiety-provoking. The last item should be the people and activities which cause you the greatest anxiety and discomfort.

Once the hierarchy has been constructed, it permits the identification of both long-term and short-term personally assessed learning goals, which range from the easiest to the most difficult. It may be found that people in relation to you fall into categories such as 'authority figures', and activities into similar groupings, such as 'learning to say no' to unreasonable requests.

Stage 3: Introduction of Systematic Assertiveness Training Skills. These skills are of two main kinds, verbal and non-verbal.
Broken Record: a skill that by calm repetition, saying what you want over and over again, teaches persistence, and permits you to ignore manipulative verbal side traps, argumentative baiting and irrelevant logic, while sticking to your desired point. This is particularly effective with persistent salesmen.

Fogging: a skill that teaches the acceptance of manipulative criticism by calmly acknowledging to your critic the probability that there may be some truth in what he or she says, yet allows you to remain your own judge of what you do. It allows you to receive criticism comfortably without becoming anxious or defensive.

Negative Assertion: a skill that teaches acceptance of your errors and faults (without having to apologize), by strongly and sympathetically agreeing with hostile or constructive criticism of your negative qualities. It permits you to look more comfortably at negative elements in your own behaviour without feeling defensive and anxious, or resorting to denial of real errors.

Negative Inquiry: a skill that teaches the active prompting of criticism in order to use the information (if helpful) or exhaust it (if manipulative), while prompting your critic to be more assertive and less dependent on manipulative ploys. It encourages the other person to express honest negative feelings and improves communication.

Workable Compromise: a skill to use whenever you feel your self-respect is not in question. Here, you offer a workable compromise to the other person. However, if the end goal involves a matter of your self-worth, there can be no compromise.

When being *assertive*, a person generally establishes good eye contact, stands or sits comfortably without fidgeting and talks in a strong, steady voice, neither shouting nor mumbling. Assertive words include 'I' statements such as 'I think', 'I feel', 'I want'; cooperative words such as 'let's', or 'we could', and empathic statements of interest such as 'what do you think', 'how do you feel'.

A *non-assertive* response is self-effacing and may be accompanied by such mannerisms as the shifting of weight, downcast eyes, a slumped body posture or a hesitant, giggly or whining voice. Non-assertive words can include qualifiers such as 'maybe', 'I wonder if you could', 'only', 'just', 'would you mind very much', 'I can't', or fillers such as 'you know', 'well', 'uh', and negators: 'it's not really important', 'it's all right', 'don't bother'.

An *aggressive* response is typically expressed by inappropriate anger or hostility which is loudly and explosively uttered. It is characterized by glaring eyes, leaning forward or pointing a finger, and an angry tone of voice. Aggressive words include threats such as 'you'd better' or 'if you don't watch out', put-downs such as 'come on', or 'you must be kidding', and evaluative comments such as 'should', 'I thought you'd know better'. Indirectly aggressive behaviour uses the language of the non-assertive response combined with the non-verbal behaviour of the aggressive mode, concentrating on body posture and angry movements.

Stage 4: Rehearsal and Role Play. This exercise draws on the essence of assertiveness training which entails personal involvement in rehearsing desired changes in behaviour. Using the individually constructed Assertive Behaviour Hierarchy (Table 2), a particular problem is selected from the top of the hierarchy. A friend, colleague or trainer can then role-play this with the trainee.

Typically, the initial performance is not assertive, and the friend or other group members in a group training section will give feedback on the verbal and non-verbal content of the individual's assertiveness. From this the individual can modify and change behaviour until he or she has found a comfortable level of assertiveness which is appropriate for them.

In the early stages of a programme, it may require more than one rehearsal and role-play session before a satisfactory level of assertiveness is attained for a particular problem. Friends and relations may help with rehearsal and role-play sessions, ensuring, of course, that they don't feature prominently in the hierarchy as 'problems' themselves.

The trainer's role in assertiveness training groups is primarily that of facilitator and coach, encouraging the identification of realistic levels of performance and encouraging the recognition and rehearsal of assertive behaviour.

Stage 5: Transfer of Behaviour 'Back Home'. When the performance is satisfactory, the behaviour is then implemented on a daily basis at work. During the training period a log of assertiveness behaviour (Table 3) is kept. Effectiveness in interactions is measured by assessing the degree of eye contact, posture, appropriate facial expression and verbal performance. The stages of the above exercise are then repeated for the next item on the hierarchy. This programme enables assertiveness in a variety of interactions, from the least threatening to the most threatening, to be improved.

The Stress Diary

In addition to identifying the activities and individuals requiring more assertive behaviour, it is important to assess those incidents and series of related incidents during the working days, weeks, and months that cause you distress. One way of doing this would be to maintain a stress diary. This should provide you with information about the type of situation, or person, that causes you the most difficulty. An awareness of this should help you to develop an *action plan* to minimize or eliminate the stress factor, or at the very

Table 3. Daily Log of Assertive Behaviour

Date	What I did	Person/people involved
_____	_____	_____
_____	_____	_____
_____	_____	_____
_____	_____	_____
_____	_____	_____
_____	_____	_____
_____	_____	_____
_____	_____	_____
_____	_____	_____

least alert you to when a stressful event (in your terms) is about to take place.

At the end of each day, for four weeks, list all the incidents, and the people involved, which caused you distress during the working day. In addition, indicate the actions taken and what you feel, in retrospect, you should have done. At the end of the month, survey the incidents and people involved which caused you the most stress, and try and pinpoint particular *types* of events and *specific* people who consistently seem to be implicated in stressful work experiences. The following Stress Identification Chart might help you to do this.

Place the *type* of event into one of the categories above, extending the list of Types of Incidents to those that are peculiar to your job and work organization. For the event involved, see if you can identify particular individuals associated with it and put their name in the appropriate columns (such as boss, subordinates,

Satisfactory aspects of performance	Aspects of performance that need improvement	Overall evaluation: excellent/good/fair/poor

colleagues, and so on). Extend these columns to incorporate additional work relationships not included in the Stress Identification Chart. Then look through all the *types of incidents* and the specific people involved, and begin to make *action plans* for the future to deal with the problem areas and the individuals concerned. For example, if you consistently find you had difficulty in dealing with your boss when it came to deadlines, think about the alternative strategies open to you to cope with this type of situation and the particular personality of the boss involved. Each incident and/or relationship can be managed if you accurately identify the problem and systematically think through the options or alternative methods of coping. Each of the coping strategies should then be ranked in terms of their *likelihood of success* in achieving your objectives, primarily to minimize future stress and accomplish your work-related tasks and goals.

Table 4. Stress Diary (four-week period)

Date	Incident	People involved
Week 1 Monday		
Tuesday		
Wednesday		
Thursday		
Friday		
Week 2 Monday		
Tuesday		
Wednesday		
Thursday		
Friday		
Week 3 Monday		
Tuesday		
Wednesday		
Thursday		
Friday		
Week 4 Monday		
Tuesday		
Wednesday		
Thursday		
Friday		

What you did

What you should have done

_____   _____

_____   _____

_____   _____

_____   _____

_____   _____

_____   _____

_____   _____

_____   _____

_____   _____

_____   _____

_____   _____

_____   _____

_____   _____

_____   _____

_____   _____

_____   _____

_____   _____

_____   _____

_____   _____

Table 5. Stress Identification Chart

Types of Incidents	Boss	Colleagues
Role-related:		
Lack of role clarity		
Conflicting role demands		
Responsibility for people		
Responsibility for things		
Overload:		
Too much work		
Too long hours		
Too much travel		
Too much detailed work		
Work interfering with:		
Home life		
Spouse		
Children		
Organizational climate:		
Too autocratic		
Too competitive		
No support		

Subordinates   **Customer/Clients**

_____   _____   _____

_____   _____   _____

_____   _____   _____

_____   _____   _____

_____   _____   _____

_____   _____   _____

_____   _____   _____

_____   _____   _____

_____   _____   _____

_____   _____   _____

_____   _____   _____

_____   _____   _____

_____   _____   _____

_____   _____   _____

_____   _____   _____

_____   _____   _____

_____   _____   _____

_____   _____   _____

Types of Incidents	Boss	Colleagues
Time pressures and deadlines:		
Unachievable deadlines		
Unnecessary time pressures		

Others:

WORKING WOMEN

Since more and more women are working, and experiencing increasing levels of stress as they attempt to manage both a career job and family, it is essential they develop a repertoire of coping skills.[4]

Obviously, the most difficult task that working women have to cope with is meeting the expectations imposed on them by the work organization, boss and family. Indeed, many feel they must excel both at work and home, that they must prove themselves competent in handling a job and the family unit. But why? Surely the most important lesson to learn is that there are inevitable conflicts between one's career and one's personal life, and that some self-management programme is necessary to keep them running smoothly and effectively. Henning and Jardim suggest one such approach.[5] They encourage their managerial women to make a list of the activities they do at work and at home, listing the hours, the tasks, the responsibilities, and the concerns they are trying to manage. They are then encouraged to examine the balance sheet and decide whether the separation of these roles (9 a.m. to 5 p.m. = worker; 5 p.m. to ? = wife/mother) is time-consuming and conflict-laden, and if so, they are advised to look for ways to blend their roles.

Following this, it would seem sensible for the working woman to begin to create action plans for dealing with the conflicts. This

Subordinates	Customer/Clients	

cannot be done alone, in isolation of the husband/boyfriend/ children; *they* must be intimately involved in the decision-making process. It would seem that the most appropriate strategy here would be a semi-formalized family role negotiation exercise, as will be outlined in Chapter 7. In addition, Frances Litman, Director of the Center for Parenting Studies at Boston's Wheelock College, tells working women to:

1 Recognize your own needs. Try and make explicit your feelings about taking on a dual role, in terms of your own family and organization.
2 Make the most of the time you do spend with the children. Women at work must make whatever time available with your children 'quality time', that is, time that is totally devoted to them, doing something enjoyable together.
3 Get the children involved in household tasks. If children can participate in the activities of the home, a stronger bond will be made between family members.
4 Agree on a fair division of household chores. This is a negotiation process between husband and wife to divide the chores in a way that takes into account the needs of both, and makes the role boundaries clear.

RE-INTEGRATING BACK HOME

'Stress at work has affected me tremendously at home. It has caused some conflict as I put an awful lot into my work and I haven't always got the energy for my husband. I think that it has caused him a lot of inner conflict too, as I have had so many problems at work and he hasn't really been able to do much. If I have had a difficult encounter, I might go home and take it out on him.

'We've found it a good thing not to talk to each other until about twenty minutes after I walk through the door, back from work. It's a strict rule of not talking. However, we may then spend anything up to an hour talking about both our work problems later in the evening. That way, we give each other emotional support regarding work stress and problems.'

CAREER MOTHER

'My eldest boy is fourteen, he's such an uncommunicative character; communications happen, but in grunts and sudden rushes of confidential information, and then silences that go on for days. He might suddenly show quite a warmth towards me when I come back from a business trip, which happens quite regularly. It seems to me to indicate that he has in some vague way been disturbed by my absence and is glad to see me back, even though he wouldn't like to say so.'

THE DOUBLE BURDEN

'My main problem is my husband's attitude to my job. He regards it as something that shouldn't intrude on the home. He has very firmly set opinions on everything. His attitude is very wearing. I find he thinks I should arrive home as fresh as anything and look after the children. I find my work physically very tiring and mentally very wearing.'

WHAT ORGANIZATIONS CAN AND SHOULD DO

Time and again we hear managing directors, personnel executives, government administrators, hospital administrators, headmasters, and others in authority roles extolling the fact that the most important resource they have is people. But when it comes right down to it, how often do organizations protect, support and nurture this most valuable asset, the human resource? Not often enough, is the simple answer. Indeed, if we treated human beings as another form of capital asset, the situation might change dramatically, as Charles Handy suggested in *Understanding Organizations*:

Salaries and benefits are really regarded as maintenance expenses – something to be kept as low as possible as long as the machine does not break down. There is no capital cost and therefore no need for depreciation. Indeed, the return on investment of most companies would look very strange if their human assets were capitalized at, say, ten times their annual maintenance cost, and depreciated over twenty years. Perhaps, one day, industrial and administrative organizations will start behaving like football clubs and charge realistic transfer fees for their key people assets.[6]

Perhaps if personnel departments or cost accountants in organizations focused more on the financial costs of the human asset, then more flexible, imaginative, and forward-looking human resource policies would be pursued. As it stands at the moment, corporate planners can choose not to concern themselves about this fickle piece of 'human machinery', discounting or depreciating it at will. Perhaps a partial solution lies with E. Flamholtz's idea that we encourage organizations to answer a series of questions about their human resources.[7] Here are some of his suggested questions, together with some of our own:

- What is the total value of your organization's human assets?
- Is it appreciating, remaining constant, or being depleted?
- How much money was spent last year to recruit and select people?
- Was this expenditure worth the cost?
- Does your organization have data on standard costs of recruitment, selection, and placement which are needed to prepare manpower budgets and to control personnel costs?
- Were the actual costs incurred last year less than, equal to, or greater than standard personnel acquisition and placement costs?
- How much money was spent last year to train and develop people?

- What was the return on your investment in training and development?
- How does this return compare with alternative investment opportunities?
- How many employees succumbed to illness or premature death?
- How much does it cost to replace these people?
- How many young people did you lose due to your promotion and/or mobility policy?
- What was the wasted 'future potential' (opportunity costs) of losing these people?
- How many women have you employed, and what has been the cost of their turnover in comparison to their male counterparts?
- Does the organization really reward managers for increasing the value of their subordinates to the firm?
- Does your promotion system accurately reflect the manager's value to the organization?
- Does your firm assess the effects of corporate strategies upon its human resources in quantitative terms?

Corporate planners and personnel policymakers must begin to ask these sorts of questions over the next decade if they are to make rational decisions about selection, training, and career development, all of which make the best possible use of human resources. The long-term payoffs may be as beneficial as the microchip or any other new technological development.

What can organizations do to cope with the increasing pressures of worklife, to minimize the costs of stress and improve the physical and mental well-being of their constituents? The rest of this chapter will focus on a number of possible corporate coping strategies which might enhance the quality of worklife.

Health Promotion and Stress Management

With the increase in 'stress' litigation, and the escalating costs of employee health care insurance, more and more American companies are providing extensive health care, stress prevention and keep-fit programmes for employees. In the UK and in Europe, however, only a few companies have flirted with stress prevention or counselling programmes. Most companies either have not tackled them seriously, or have abandoned their efforts. In addition, many company doctors and personnel executives who see the problems of stress at work have found it difficult to implement stress management courses and programmes because senior managers feel that 'stress is none of our business', or 'employees should be able to cope on their own', or 'our responsibility is to make profits for our shareholders, not to mollycoddle our employees'.

Even if organizations doubt that they bear responsibility for employee health care or stress prevention at work, they should see the cost-saving argument in terms of lost work days, absenteeism, poor performance, premature death, and retraining. In the US, the cost arguments and the legal implications of *cumulative trauma* have weighed heavily in favour of primary prevention within companies. US organizations have used a number of different approaches towards stress prevention or health care: the provision of keep-fit facilities on site, dietary control, relaxation and exercise classes, stress or psychological counselling, or some combination of these.

The health promotion and stress prevention schemes are as colourfully labelled as they are idiosyncratic in their orientation: 'wellness programme', 'treatment of chemically dependent employees', 'employee assistance programme', 'lifestyle change programme' and the like.[8] It has been reported that the New York Telephone Company's wellness programme (that is, cardiovascular fitness) saved the organization $2.7 million in absence and treatment costs in one year alone. The giant copper corporation, Kennecott Corporation, introduced a counselling programme for employees in distress. This produced a drop in absenteeism of nearly 60 per cent in one year and a 55 per cent reduction in medical costs.

Pepsico Inc. has created a comprehensive physical fitness programme at its world headquarters at Purchase, New York. Facilities include a fully fitted gymnasium, with a sauna, an electrical treadmill, a striking bag (not moulded in the shape of the chief executive!), stationary bicycles, whirlpool baths, showers, and massage facilities. In addition, employees have a 1.15 mile running track which circles the H Q complex. This programme is under the supervision of a full-time physical therapist and medical physician. Tailor-made exercise programmes are designed for any interested employee by the physical therapist or doctor. Although this facility was originally planned for senior executives, it is now used by all employees on a voluntary basis. The corporate H Q is located in an attractive park-like setting providing an atmosphere which encourages physical fitness. Also provided are regular sessions in aerobic dancing, yoga, as well as diet training to meet the needs of individual employees, and so on.

In West Germany, the chemical company B A S F A G, twice a year takes a group of thirty-six executives away from their offices for a two-week training session in personal health. They swim, jog, take saunas, stick to a well-planned diet, and are encouraged to take part in relaxation sessions such as yoga and transcendental meditation. By taking executives away for an intensive health programme, management hopes to encourage them to adopt more positive attitudes towards physical and mental health for themselves.

In Canada, Canada Life Assurance Co. and North American Life Assurance Co. participated jointly in a research project to see what effects a keep-fit programme would have on their managers. In all, 1,125 managers from both companies were enrolled into a systematic physical fitness course in their H Q gymnasium. The companies found several interesting results. Firstly, there was a drop in absenteeism of 22 per cent which, if translated across the whole company, could mean a saving of some $200,000 year. Secondly, they found a 3 per cent rise in productivity in the exercising group as opposed to the unfit one. In addition, they found that the keep-fit managers had a significantly more positive attitude towards work and reported better relationships with their bosses and subordinates.

Converse Corporation in Wilmington did a variation on the keep-fit theme by providing a voluntary twelve-week relaxation programme for their employees. Over 140 volunteered and were compared to sixty-three non-volunteers who were selected randomly. The volunteers agreed to keep daily records for twelve weeks and to have their blood pressure measured. In addition, their general health and job performance were assessed during the experimental period. The results indicated that not only was a relaxation training break feasible within normal working hours, but that it led to improvements in general health, job performance and well-being. In addition, there was a significant decrease in the blood pressure of managers from the start to the finish of the training.

Perhaps the best kind of approach a company can follow is the example of the engineering company Emhart Corporation. Managers were concerned about the health of their employees, but were cautious about investing large sums of money into a fitness programme that their employees might not use. So they first surveyed their staff about their attitudes to a company keep-fit programme, and on the basis of a positive response built a low-cost gymnasium. Then, after it became clear that the employees were using it regularly, they expanded the facilities (and hired experienced exercise instructors). After a year of operation they realized that the demand was so great that they built a jogging track. It was a step-by-step approach, with each preceding one justifying the next.

By far the most comprehensive and best researched of these programmes was undertaken by Control Data Corporation, one of the largest American computer companies. Like many major US firms, it now 'self-insures' – covering its employees directly and therefore has control of its own health care costs. Its programme is called STAYWELL and is provided for the 22,000 Control Data employees and their spouses in fourteen American cities as a 'free corporate benefit'. It has five components which encourage giving up smoking, weight control, cardiovascular fitness, stress management and improved diet (particularly, cutting down on cholesterol, salt and sugar). Each employee goes through three steps:

1 A confidential health-risk profile or screening is conducted. There is a comprehensive physical examination, but the employee also gives information on lifestyle and health behaviour (like smoking and drinking). This information is kept entirely confidential to the medical and nursing staff.
2 The employee attends an 'interpretation session'. Here he gets personal results and action plans to reduce specific health risks.

3 Finally, the employee selects the appropriate course (on weight control or on stress management, for example), given his or her risk profile. Employee enrolment in the various Control Data Corporation schemes has ranged from 65 to 95 per cent at different sites throughout the US. Management and blue-collar workers participate equally.

But what is the outcome? The evidence is startling. Control Data explored the average health care costs claims of their employees, and their hospital stays, and discovered:

- Employees who were encouraged to quit smoking spent half the number of days in hospital, and had 20 per cent less health care costs, compared with smokers.
- Those that underwent exercise training had 30 per cent fewer claims, and spent half the number of days in hospital, compared with the sedentary group.
- Most revealing of all, those employees who entered the cardiovascular fitness programme, and reduced their hypertension levels, had less than half the health care costs of those who did not.
- In addition, when Control Data checked out the employees they rated 'most at risk' versus those 'least at risk' in terms of health habits (weight, stress, fitness, nutrition and smoking), they found that the high-risk employees were twice as likely to be absent from work due to sickness, and to be half as productive, as the low-risk or physically fit group.

In almost all of these health promotion programmes, there is a strong emphasis on the management and prevention of stress. This US orientation to health promotion and stress management is beginning to take hold in the UK. There are a number of UK companies or affiliates of foreign companies who are actively involved in this development, such as Control Data (UK), Shell Chemicals, Johnson and Johnson, and Air Canada (UK). One of the most recent and innovative developments is the Post Office, which has introduced stress counsellors in two main metropolitan regions. The counsellors will not only help individuals cope with stress in the workplace, but also identify sources of organizational stress that may be causing the problems. On the basis of any problems identified, they will work with the regional postal authority in planning and initiating organizational change, in redesigning jobs or whatever is necessary to correct the basic or structural problems within the organization. They are also carrying out a simultaneous evaluation of the effectiveness of the counselling in two control cities, which will help them focus on the most effective aspects of the stress-counselling role. This will enable the Post Office to refine the nature of the role and help in the further introduction of this concept throughout the postal service.

Regardless of the moral or humanistic arguments, from the point of view of costs and benefits protecting the human asset should be a major concern of any enterprise. The General Motors Corporation spends about $2,000 a year per employee on health care insurance, and over $1.3 billion overall (in 1978 alone), which was a thirty-fold increase on 1960.

Stress awareness in Bosses

Auden, in his poem *The Unknown Citizen*, wrote, 'Was he free? Was he happy? The question is absurd: had anything been wrong, we should certainly have heard.' But can or should we rely exclusively on informal hearsay filtering through the organization about the well-being of one of our fellow employees? Stressful behaviour all too frequently can be disguised or covered up in some acceptable form, at least in its initial stages. It is important, with the increasing pressures of organizational life, to provide managers with some awareness of how stress can be manifested in themselves and others (subordinates and colleagues). Once a manager is aware of the symptoms of stress, particularly in respect of himself and his subordinates, he or she is in a better position to do something about them, either at the level of encouraging the person to participate in some form of stress-reduction training programme or in modifying the job stress factors.

This training programme could not only include creating an awareness of the possible stress manifestations, but also sessions where the managers look at themselves and share with their trainee colleagues the way in which they react to pressure, and the events, people and organizational characteristics that they feel are responsible. Understanding one's own and other people's reactions to stress in such sessions can prove invaluable in the work environment. These types of programmes should probably be composed of a cross-section of employees from different departments, divisions or sections, which would help dispel the prejudice that is still inherent in attitudes towards stress problems.

When the norms in a company are changed to acknowledge and accept the reality of stress, the process of managing it – as opposed to eliminating it, which is probably neither possible nor desirable – will be easier and probably more effective. One of the most efficacious ways of preventing, rather than coping with, the pressures of working in organizations is by establishing support systems among staff: management can encourage employees to help one another, share their concerns, reorganize work schedules and tasks to aid those in greatest need, acknowledge that family circumstances can affect performance and offer help to their employees or subordinate managers or bosses who are experiencing difficult home problems, and so on. The creation of support groups at different levels of the organization could be done with the help of management development advisers, who would act as an informal counselling service to all managers. This should not be just a mechanism for dealing with immediate problems or individuals who are manifestly 'at the end of their tether', but rather a group that meets regularly. An on-going group is likely to see the development of problems and potential stress agents, and can help individuals to recognize them and plan their activities to minimize or eliminate them before it is too late.

As a philosophical sidenote we can ask whether competition among managers is always necessary or healthy for an organization. Indeed, a recent study undertaken by University of Texas researchers has found that the most competitive individuals are not necessarily the ones who achieve the most. Success is predicated much more on the desire to work hard and a drive towards 'achieving personal standards of excellence' than on aggression or competition. Many more people are beginning to feel that competitive and cut-throat behaviour at work not only leads to stress-related illness and job dissatisfaction but also to lower overall organizational productivity.[9]

HELPING DUAL-EARNER FAMILIES AND WORKING WOMEN

With the large number of women entering the workforce over the next decade, indeed, with the United Kingdom slowly becoming a dual-career nation, it is incumbent on organizations to develop human resources policies that will minimize the current stresses and strains which are experienced by both men and women of two-earner families.[10]

One way in which an organization can help them is to recognize some of the difficulties of working women and begin to provide the necessary support. For example, New England Mutual Life Insurance Company discovered that 70 per cent of their female employees who became pregnant left the firm permanently. They decided to do something to help those who wanted to work and raise a family concurrently, and by the late 1970s only 30 per cent of the mothers-to-be stopped working. They devised a series of seminars for their working mothers to attend during the lunch hour, and this was offered to over 2,300 employees. These seminars explored a wide variety of problems experienced by dual-career parents, as well as allowing a high level of participation so that those present could share their difficulties. And most importantly, they tried to get working mothers to make explicit their guilt feelings about not playing out the traditional mother role in the home. Although such an experience is likely to be beneficial, it is important that companies also acknowledge the reality of dual-career families and accommodate to them with practical measures. What is truly needed is the following policy changes.

Flexible Working Arrangements

There are a wide range of flexible working arrangements that organizations can provide for their male and female employees to accommodate to changing family patterns. *Flexitime* is obviously one good example. In order for working mothers or fathers to meet the psychological responsibilities associated with their children's education, or indeed, to free themselves of the guilt of not fulfilling traditional roles *vis-à-vis* children, many parents feel that they must take their children to school and pick them up. This is very difficult to accomplish under the current 9 a.m. to 5 p.m. (or later) working hours, and would be made much easier under flexitime conditions – as long as they applied to both husband and wife. And why shouldn't flexitime be extended to school vacation times? Many dual-career parents are concerned about arrangements for their children during the summer months when they are at home. There are several ways of coping with this problem: allowing the wife or husband to have a lighter load during these months; allowing them to build up a backlog of working time during other months to relieve them during these months; providing facilities on site during the summer months for young children (perhaps by using university students training in the field of primary education), or some combination of these.

Another flexible working arrangement would be more part-time work in a variety of different forms: limiting the number of days a week, or hours in a day, or indeed shortening the working week by allowing individuals to work a forty-hour week in three or four days. This last suggestion is growing in popularity; a dual-career husband and wife can, by careful planning, be able to manage their domestic and work arrangements between them. In 1972, an American Management Association survey estimated that between 700 and 1,000 firms of over 100,000 employees were on a four-day, forty-hour week in the US. By 1975, the number of firms grew to 3,000 covering more than 1 million workers. Today, the figure is close to 3 million workers. Indeed, many firms are moving to a three-day, thirty-eight-hour week without decline in productivity and job satisfaction.[11]

Organizations can also provide crèches or nursery facilities in the workplace. There is an increasing growth of these in many of the 'advanced thinking' organizations. Many educationalists and psychologists have felt this is a good idea because it provides the mother or father with the opportunity of seeing their children some time during working hours. A less satisfactory solution would be community-based nurseries, but these may be necessary for those who work for small companies or who are self-employed. The benefits that organizations could derive from the introduction of the industrial kibbutzim seem to be obvious – less time taken off work, to name but one – and it is surprising that more companies have not followed suit.

Parental Leave

It is obvious that many women at work who are preparing to have a family need some sense of security about their jobs. In this respect it seems only sensible to have reasonable maternity leave with a guaranteed right to return to work and financial security during the leave period. Most countries in the European Economic Community have guarantees against dismissal during pregnancy and a guarantee of paid maternity leave (usually up to six months and between six and twelve months in many Eastern European countries). Some countries also have guarantees of the right to return to work either immediately following the paid maternity leave or to receive unpaid leave for some prearranged period (in some cases up to two or three years).

Parental leave is particularly important in the changing circumstances of the family. Few organizations in Western countries provide this contemporary innovation, but many will have to consider it in the near future or soon face an uncontrolled absenteeism problem. Dual-career families will increasingly need the flexibility of short-leave periods, and the provision of leave for both men and women should help to ease the problem.

Working at Home

With the advent of the microprocessor revolution, it should become increasingly easier for husbands and wives in certain types of jobs to work at home. The need for a central workplace should decrease quite dramatically over the next decade or two. Already, employees can take home a computer terminal or a minicomputer itself to carry out many of the tasks that once they were only able to do in a centralized work environment. In order to be able to do this, organizations will have to rid themselves of their deep-rooted, nefarious suspicion of their employees, that is, that the latter will take every opportunity to exploit their employer and work as little as possible; and that only by overseeing them will work get done! Indeed, it is this very control that has made the process of work for many unsatisfying and has encouraged the compartmentalization of work and home life to the detriment of both. As sociologist C. Wright Mills once said, 'Each day men sell little pieces of themselves in order to try and buy them back each night and weekend with little pieces of fun.'

Some organizations may one day realize that they do not necessarily need a centralized workplace at all. For the time being, however, work organizations ought to explore the variety of jobs that could easily be done at home and provide this degree of flexibility to their employees. At the very least, it is worth an experiment!

Long Hours

All too often organizations create a norm of long hours. Employees are made to feel guilty if they leave by five o'clock in the afternoon, and they are subtly encouraged to work into the early evening. This can dramatically affect the activities of the family, taking away 'quality time' that the individual could spend with children and spouse. Is it necessary to work sixty hours a week? What is the organization really saying when it inculcates this norm? Is it merely a mechanism for the company to obtain a show of commitment? Are there not better ways to do this than create unnecessary conflicts between home and work? Indeed, one would have thought that the use of long hours might produce the effect contrary to the one desired, that is, might create in the employee's spouse and family an antagonism towards the organization and what it represents. The organization will then be seen as the 'great intruder' in the family home, the unfeeling, uncaring employer who takes the husband/father or wife/mother away from family activities at will. The questions that organizations should ask themselves about particular employees are:

- Does this employee need to work beyond the forty-hour week? If so, why?
- How might this be affecting the person's work and family life? If it is adversely affecting both, what can be done to minimize its effect or what support could be provided?

- Could the individual's working hours be altered flexibly to allow more quality time at home during busy periods or projects?

Smoothing the Way for Women

Many women who have played the traditional family 'caring' role need particular help if they are to change the pattern of their marriage and fulfil a more dual role. One problem these women may face after many years away from work is lack of confidence and the feeling that they are out of date (they may actually be out of date). It is in the interest of employers and the wider community to provide opportunities for these women to be brought up to date with current developments. This might best be done by professional associations or by work organizations providing up-dating courses for ex-employees who have temporarily left employment to raise a family. As M. P. Fogarty has suggested, 'The important thing in the interests of both employers and of young mothers themselves is to minimize the interruption of a highly qualified woman's career and to keep her as closely in touch as possible with her particular world of work.'[12] Any help the organization can give its former employees in maintaining their skills may pay off greatly in the future, not only in terms of 'goodwill', but also in reducing costs of retraining or initial training of new staff. As for the need to increase confidence, this can be accomplished during the up-dating activity or by specialized courses prior to retraining or up-dating.

Providing Career Opportunities to Female Managers

In addition to helping the dual-career woman cope within her domestic and work environments, it is important for organizations to encourage women to enter management and then provide them with career opportunities once there. Increasingly, companies are providing 'affirmative action officers' or some equivalent personnel role to try and adhere to the spirit of Equal Opportunities Commission requirements. These people are responsible for examining the existing imbalances in the organization and recommending what can be done to make it easier for women to take up managerial positions. Changing managerial recruitment policy, providing facilities for working mothers, changing male-biased company literature which might put off a prospective female manager are all possible actions. An economist, S. Ekberg-Jordan, has suggested a number of organizational changes that are needed to support the careers of female managers:

1 *Career planning and counselling.* Because of the special needs and circumstances of some women, it is necessary to plan and counsel women on their short-range job prospects and their long-term career goals. This may include a period of retraining or up-dating at some suitable time in their careers, as well as providing a periodic mechanism for feedback on *their* current perform-ance.

2 *Providing senior management sponsorship.* To encourage and help support women managers, a system of sponsorship within the organization can be useful in the corporate jungle. This role would entail helping the female manager to meet colleagues, to better understand the organization's informal procedures and customs, and to acquaint her with any other peculiarities of corporate life (e.g. myths about the company, its history, etc.).

3 *Helping male managers to come to terms with female managers.* To establish training programmes within the company to get male and female managers to share their perceptions, stereotypes, myths and feelings about one another, and particularly about the role of women in management. The goal here is to try to change male managers' views of their female counterparts, and to encourage them to be more supportive and less threatened.

4 *The creation of informal support networks for all women man-agers.* This may be particularly helpful while women are still very much in the minority in the organization, but less necessary as they begin to establish themselves in larger numbers and throughout the organization.[13]

Flexible Working Life

As organizations begin to plan for the long-term future of their human resources, they will require a 'new look', a more flexible approach to working life. Fred Best of the National Commission for Manpower Policy in Washington, D.C. describes this as 'an entirely revolutionary *flexilife* timetable for the society of the future'. In this New World, it is not hard to imagine a dramatic change in the life cycles of most individuals. During the early years of work, when the individual is single and unmarried, he or she is likely to work long hours per week to show their commitment to the organization. When the individual gets married and has children, more flexible work and leisure periods will have to be negotiated, with the likely outcome of a shorter working week, parental leaves, and other arrangements. With the children grown, there may be a shift back to longer working weeks but also longer periods of leisure, as well as occasional sabbatical periods. During the 'empty nest' stage, however, when the children are gone and the individual is approaching early retirement, there is likely to be a gradual process of withdrawal; this can mean a gradual reduction of the working week, longer periods of planned leisure, and possibly the development of other skills needed for alternative, perhaps less demanding, work or community service in the future.

The future of work and leisure will depend on technological and social development over the next couple of decades. But will this change be continuous? Handy suggests that 'in conditions of continuous change we project the status quo into the future, we run the graphs up the charts, multiplying or dividing by appropriate amounts what we do today to meet the requirements of tomorrow'.[14] The process of planning is predicated by most people on the assumptions of continuous change. On the other hand, because of the technological and social developments over the last decade, change in the future is likely to be discontinuous, when today's methods, attitudes, and ways of living will not work tomorrow. As Handy emphasizes, 'How many blacksmiths coped with discontinuous change in their industry by becoming motor mechanics?' While planning can work in a situation of continuous change, it will not work in circumstances of discontinuous change. What is needed in the future of discontinuous change are 'lateral thinkers', a different approach to viewing the world, and an appreciation that things may not be like they have been. Edward De Bono in his book *Opportunities*, summed this up beautifully:

Imagine that you are attracted by tall blondes, and that you are at a party and spot a tall blonde at the other end of the room. The room is crowded. You move about the room asking your friends whether any of them knows the blonde well enough to introduce you. It is a tiresome process. Yet had you looked around you before starting off on the quest you would have seen that standing just behind you was an even more attractive blonde conversing with a good friend of yours. The moral is that opportunities may not be difficult to see in themselves but they remain impossible to see if we happen to be looking in the wrong direction.[15]

A more flexible approach to one's work and life planning is also an aid to the increasing problems experienced by many professional men and women in middle life, quaintly termed 'the midlife crisis'. In a sample of over 2,000 male and female executives, a psychologist found that 80 per cent of those who reach middle life experience a personal crisis, which has implications for work and private life.[16] Indeed, Ivan Turgenev, in his novel *Fathers and Sons*, highlighted this process through his character, Pavel: 'To Nikolai there remained the sense of a well spent life; Pavel on the contrary, a solitary bachelor, was entering upon that indefinite twilight period of regrets that are akin to hopes and hopes that are akin to regrets, when youth is over, while old age has not yet come.'

Planning for your mid-life crisis might seem somewhat pessimistic, but life planning which builds in flexibility and an acknowledgment of the realities of the human condition can only help. Psychologist T. Lidz leaves us with an interesting observation:

In the tradition from adolescence to early adulthood, the individual has become committed to a way of life; he has now lived it and is now mature – or is unlikely ever to become mature. Now approaching the divide, he looks back and also tries to prognosticate on the basis of this experience. Perhaps he will try to climb still higher, change course while he still can, or decide upon which path of descent is safest. Whether a person makes the most of the opportunity available or whether he begins to die slowly depends . . .[17]

This depends not only on the organization or on the other people we live and work with, but on ourselves. The individual must take responsibility for his own development.

CONCLUSION

Many of the issues and suggestions in this chapter are not new to anyone working in organizations. The workplace can provide a great sense of achievement and satisfaction or a feeling of failure and dissatisfaction. It is important for the future of an effective and less stressful worklife that organizations, in the public as well as the private sector, begin to think about their structures, policies and working practices with regard to their human resources. As Alastair Mant suggests in his book *The Rise and Fall of the British Manager*, 'a great deal of what wants doing in this naughty world seems to be reasonably obvious to men and women of goodwill and common sense everywhere. But we have not, it seems, mastered the trick of creating the intervening institutions that help us to get things done. We have instead a fantasy of freedom and a distrust of institutional restraint and "red tape" which ultimately binds us. We rush headlong from analysis to action, without stopping *en route* to build sound constitutional structures to support our endeavours.'[18] Setting up appropriate personnel policies to support, encourage, and develop individuals throughout the organizational hierarchy, therefore, is what we ought to be aiming for. We must view employees as individuals who have needs, personalities, and commitments outside the confines of organizational life, and begin to realize (and put into practice) that the performance, efficiency, and satisfaction of an employee is linked to his or her total life experience.

If we can only keep the words of A. Kornhauser once again in mind, we should be on the right track:

Mental health is not so much a freedom from specific frustrations as it is an overall balanced relationship to the world, which permits a person to maintain a realistic, positive belief in himself and his purposeful activities. Insofar as his entire job and life situation facilitate and support such feelings of adequacy, inner security, and meaningfulness of his existence, it can be presumed that his mental health will tend to be good. What is important in a negative way is not any single characteristic of his situation but everything that deprives the person of purpose and zest, that leaves him with negative feelings about himself, with anxieties, tensions, a sense of lostness, emptiness, and futility.[19]

Chapter 7

COPING WITH LIFE STRESS

'If what you're doing is making you sick, stop doing it.'

Abraham Maslow

If you have read the preceding six chapters, and not skipped ahead due to your 'hurry sickness', you probably have a fairly good idea of the sources of stress in your personal life. You may have identified personality characteristics and life situations that make you more stress-prone, and may have recognized ways to cope better with stress at work. This final chapter will help translate your personal 'stress vulnerability profile' into coping action. As we promised in Chapter 1, you may learn how to deal better with stress and, hopefully, become more effective at coping.

KNOW THYSELF

Although this chapter will provide many aids and techniques to reduce stress levels, it is the authors' belief that any success in dealing with life stress must begin with self-knowledge. Through the exercises in this book, you may have learned more about yourself in terms of Type A or Type B behaviour, your own locus of control and the degree to which life events have affected your stress level. For many people, further exploration may be required. It will be important to understand whether your high stress level is primarily generated by personal conflicts or from a need to create more balance in your life. For most people, there is no one problem that must be solved; neither is there one answer. As discussed throughout this book, poor coping with stress usually involves many factors, including the individual's personality and coping strategies, life events encountered and degree of social support.

While there are many things an individual cannot control, such as the loss of a loved one, many things most certainly can be managed or at least modified by the individual. Often, self-knowledge brings the awareness that an individual must alter his or her perceptions, behaviour, lifestyle or personal situation in order to cope effectively with stress. For some people, the only changes required will be simple ones, such as incorporating more relaxation into daily life. For others, a change in work or home arrangements may be necessary. Of course, a person can always choose not to make any changes, and to continue as usual and hope for the best. The person who refuses to make changes in his or her life is really *choosing* to endure the present situation, rather than trying to improve things. Change is difficult and taking responsibility is difficult. But the rewards, in terms of personal happiness and effectiveness, may be worth the effort involved.

Wayne Dyer, in his book *Your Erroneous Zones*, talks about self-immobilization as the force of resistance to change in our lives; this can range from total inaction to mild indecision and hesitancy. He argues that we must cut through this unhealthy, yet understandable resistance in order to release our 'potential for happiness'. He urges individuals to focus on those aspects of lifestyle that may create immobility, and suggests a number of possible behaviours that reflect this state:

> You are immobilized when . . .
> You can't talk lovingly to your spouse and children though you want to.
> You can't work on a project that interests you.
> You don't make love and would like to.
> You sit in the house all day and brood.
> You don't play golf, tennis, or other enjoyable activities, because of a leftover gnawing feeling.
> You can't introduce yourself to someone who appeals to you.
> You avoid talking to someone when you realize that a simple gesture would improve your relationship.
> You can't sleep because something is bothering you.
> Your anger keeps you from thinking clearly.
> You say something abusive to someone you love.
> Your face is twitching, or you are so nervous that you don't function in the way you would prefer.[1]

Dyer believes an individual must be able to identify the problem areas or lifestyle patterns that are preventing him or her from achieving life goals, and then 'cut through the lifetime of emotional red tape' by changing behaviour and redesigning these patterns. What Dyer warns against – and this is a cardinal rule – is blaming any circumstance or other person for failures or an unsatisfying mode of living. People must 'own up', take responsibility and choose a more satisfying way to live. As George Bernard Shaw put it in his play *Mrs Warren's Profession*, 'People are always blaming their circumstances for what they are. I don't believe in circumstances. The people who get on in this world are the people who get up and look for the circumstances they want, and if they can't find them, make them.'

CHOOSING HOW TO LIVE

To some stress researchers, the decision to choose a more satisfying lifestyle must begin with a basic decision to live. Martin Shaffer, in his book *Life After Stress*, states that the stress-resilient person has 'decided to live. This person is not ambivalent about living or dying. He embraces life – at home, at work, or at play.' He believes that most people do not have a firm desire to live or die; in fact, they tend to lean towards self-destruction. Evidence of this is illustrated by their smoking, drinking, over-eating or similar destructive activities. Shaffer suggests that we should ask ourselves, 'Do I want to live?' until this question can be answered with a positive 'Yes!' If the answer is 'No', we should seek professional help to determine the reasons behind this answer, which is seldom a rational one. Shaffer suggests that once the will to live is firmly established, each of us can develop a list of positive reasons for living and a description of how we want to live, in the categories of physical well-being and health, personal relationships, work, spiritual and creative growth, relaxation and play.[2]

Advice abounds on how to live, full of descriptions of just which qualities constitute a 'healthy, creative' lifestyle. Not all of these ideals will meet the needs or wants of everyone. However, for those who desire some guidelines to what might be considered as 'reasonable living patterns', Karl Albrecht provides a rich behavioural description in his book *Stress and the Manager*.[3] Table 1 shows Albrecht's description of the low-stress versus high-stress lifestyle.

The table shows that many elements of the low-stress lifestyle are ways of living based on common sense, such as eating well and using alcohol sparingly or not at all. Other elements, such as the development of 'escape routes' and a lifestyle with little role conflict are more creative approaches.

MANAGING YOUR OWN LIFESTYLE

You may have determined that your lifestyle is not providing you what you need in terms of resilience to stress and of relief. Before providing you with suggestions on how to change certain stress-inducing behaviours, it is important that you determine *for yourself* exactly where you want these changes to lead. The exercise of 'life planning', in addition to clarifying your direction and goals, can actually help you feel more in control of yourself and your life.

One such exercise has been developed by Bill Pfeiffer and John Jones.[4] There are three parts to this exercise. The first part is aimed at answering the question, 'where am I now?' in three areas – your career, your personal life (friends and family) and your personal fulfilment, and it proceeds as follows:

1 Draw a graph or life-line, which can be straight or curved, that depicts the trend of the past, present and future of your career. Place an X to show where you are now. Then write a brief explanation of the career line you have drawn, highlighting the high points and the low points.
2 Repeat the procedure to create a life-line for your personal life with highs and lows.
3 Repeat again to create a personal fulfilment life-line.

This part of the exercise should give you some idea of where you've been, where you are now and where you are likely to go. The future aspects of each line may reflect either your hopes for where you ideally would go or where you think you are likely to end up (although you would rather not).

Table 1. High- and Low-stress Lifestyle

Stressful Lifestyle	Low-stress Lifestyle
Individual experiences chronic, unrelieved stress.	Individual accepts 'creative' stress for distinct periods of challenging activity.
Becomes trapped in one or more continuing stressful situations. Struggles with stressful interpersonal relationships (family, spouse, lover, boss, co-workers, etc.).	Has 'escape routes' allowing occasional detachment and relaxation. Asserts own rights and needs; negotiates low-stress relationships of mutual respect; selects friends carefully and establishes relationships that are nourishing and not harmful.
Engages in distasteful, dull, toxic, or otherwise unpleasant and unrewarding work.	Engages in challenging, satisfying, worthwhile work that offers intrinsic rewards for accomplishment.
Experiences continual time stress: too much to be done in available time.	Maintains a well-balanced and challenging workload; overloads and crises are balanced by 'breather' periods.
Worries about potentially unpleasant up-coming events.	Balances threatening events with worthwhile goals and positive events to look forward to.
Has poor health habits (e.g. eating, smoking, liquor, lack of exercise, poor level of physical fitness). Life activities are 'lopsided' or unbalanced (e.g. preoccupied with one activity such as work, social activities, making money, solitude, or physical activities).	Maintains high level of physical fitness, eats well, uses alcohol and tobacco not at all or sparingly. Life activities are balanced: individual invests energies in a variety of activities, which, in the aggregate, bring feelings of satisfaction (e.g. work, social activities, recreation, solitude, cultural pursuits, family and close relationships).
Finds it difficult to just 'have a good time', relax and enjoy momentary activities. Experiences sexual activities as unpleasant, unrewarding, or socially programmed (e.g. by manipulation, 'one-upping').	Finds pleasure in simple activities, without feeling a need to justify playful behaviour. Enjoys a full and exuberant sex life, with honest expression of sexual appetite.

Sees life as a serious, difficult situation; little sense of humour.	Enjoys life, on the whole; can laugh at him/herself; has a well-developed and well-exercised sense of humour.
Conforms to imprisoning, punishing social roles.	Lives a relatively role-free life; is able to express natural needs, desires, and feelings without apology.
Accepts high-pressure or stressful situations passively; suffers in silence.	Acts assertively to re-engineer pressure situations whenever possible; renegotiates impossible deadlines; avoids being placed in unnecessary pressure situations; manages time effectively.

Source: Karl Albrecht, *Stress and the Manager* (New Jersey: Prentice-Hall, 1979) 107–8.

The second part of the exercise asks you to find out 'who am I?' by writing down up to twenty career adjectives which most accurately describe you in your work, such as ambitious, trustworthy, nonchalant, and so on. Then write down a similar list of adjectives for your personal life and personal fulfilment.

Divide each group of adjectives into three categories: positive, negative and neutral. This regrouping can provide you with an awareness of your positive and negative traits in three major aspects of your life.

In the third part of the exercise, ask yourself where you want to be. List up to ten ideal attainments in each of the three main life areas – career, personal life and personal fulfilment. Goals might include 'I want to become self-employed', or 'I want to re-establish closeness with my husband', or 'I want to face my need for alcohol'.

Then assign priority values to the ideals within each of the three groups, using the following scale: 4 = of very great importance; 3 = of great importance; 2 = of moderate importance; and 1 = of little importance.

Finally, combine all the ideals into one group and rank them again, using the same scoring system. The combined list should reflect the relative importance of specific goals, whether they involve your career, personal life or personal fulfilment. This then gives you information about your ideal goals in life. You are now equipped with a launching pad for life planning.

A way to begin your planning efforts would be to select five or so of the highest rated goals and establish a programme to achieve them, one by one. You will need to think out the behavioural, emotional and practical strategies for each goal. Such an effort is not easy, but by writing out your goals and strategies, you may see solutions you had not conceived before. This process may be easier if you work with someone else, with whom you could share your goals and eventual progress. If so, deliberately seek out a trusted colleague, relative or friend. In order to reward yourself for your progress, design specific strategies and objectives that can be measured, rather than just vague ideals. For example, if closeness with a spouse is a goal, a strategy might be to plan one evening out together each week. The initiation of small changes can one by one lead to the larger life goals established in your plan.

By analysing the life goals you have established in the three areas of career, personal life and personal fulfilment, you may see that the time and energy you have in the past given to one area is far greater than that given the other two. Many professionals, for example, may find they have developed their careers to the neglect of their home life, friendships, and personal needs for health and creativity. The establishment of concrete goals in each of the three areas can be a first step towards restoring balance and wholeness to life.

The concept of life planning involves a basic idea: setting goals and objectives helps give direction and a sense of control of time, a precious and limited commodity. Once you have worked through the life planning exercises, the same process of setting specific goals and priorities can be applied to monthly, weekly and daily planning. Although the creation of a time management programme is beyond the scope of this book, any such programme will grow out of the basic process of setting goals and prioritizing, as well as eliminating those tasks which are superfluous and learning to protect your time by saying 'no'. An excellent guide to time management can be found in *How to Get Control of Your*

Time and Your Life by Alan Lakein.[5] He recommends using a written list of things to do, with every item on the list receiving a priority rating such as high, medium or low. By concentrating on the top-priority items first, and then dealing with the remainder in order, you can gain a better sense of accomplishment and control.

MAKING CHANGES

Much of the remainder of this chapter will examine ways you can work to alter stress-inducing behaviour and situations, and will also offer suggestions on how to add positive elements to your life to help you resist stress. Making changes can seem overwhelming at first. But remember, stress is not some all-powerful force in your life that cannot be resisted. Rather, your life is most likely full of small and large stress responses that either can be altered or, at the least, balanced with other, more positive experiences, such as relaxation. Before you consider the suggestions offered below, it may be worthwhile to examine any feelings of resistance you harbour to the idea that your life can change. Sometimes it is helpful to consider someone else you know who is experiencing undue amounts of stress. Perhaps you have observed a family member or friend who is suffering from time pressures or other stress factors. It may be relatively easy for you to see how a few changes in that person's life, such as getting up half an hour earlier to get a better grip on the day, or learning to say 'no' when demands become too great, could improve the situation. You perhaps have even offered a suggestion to that person, only to be told, 'Yes, that's a good idea, but . . .' Suggestions are often greeted with a variety of responses, all of which boil down to, 'I can't'. Depressed people, especially, may find it difficult to see options, even if they are pointed out by others. Psychologists recognize the inability to see options as a key characteristic of depression. When you consider the suggestions offered below, ask yourself if you are responding with, 'I can't'. Force yourself to consider each idea and seriously try to see if you can change your response to 'I will'.

MONITORING YOURSELF

In earlier chapters, you have examined personality characteristics, life events, coping strategies, and work and family situations that may give rise to stress in your life. You have also been able to consider the toll that stress may be taking on you physically and mentally. However, as part of an effort to apply this knowledge to your life, you may want to begin monitoring when you are actually subject to stress responses. You can soon learn to recognize your own personal stress warning signals – such as headaches, stomach pains, muscle tension, or a strong desire to escape from a situation. A stress diary, in which you note responses such as anxiety or depression and the situations in which they occur, can help you uncover patterns in your life. Or you might choose to devote a space of a few hours or days to analysing specifically when and where you feel tense or stressful. Putting these thoughts down on paper can help crystallize your thinking. Periodically setting aside time to analyse the sources of stress and balance in your life can become a tremendously rewarding habit. Also, becoming aware of your body's responses to stress and anxiety can begin to provide valuable clues to what's happening in your life.

MANAGING TYPE A BEHAVIOUR

If you determined from the questionnaire in Chapter 3 that you lean towards Type A behaviour, you may want to consider suggestions aimed at managing this behaviour. Friedman and Rosenman, the originators of the link between Type A behaviour and high incidences of coronary heart disease, don't maintain that this behaviour should be changed, but rather *managed*, to reduce the health-risk implications involved. In addition to the life-prolonging motivation needed to deal with Type A behaviour, it should be noted that at least one research project has indicated that successful professional men are more similar to the Type B personality than Type A. In this study, the most successful types were not hard-driving, aggressive and competitive; rather, they were relaxed and possessed a warmth that attracted others.[6]

In their book *Type A Behavior and Your Heart*, Friedman

and Rosenman recommend a number of 'drills against hurry sickness', which they maintain work for their Type A patients:[7]

1 Try to restrain yourself from being the centre of attention by constantly talking. Force yourself to listen to others. 'Begin in your advocational hours to listen quietly to the conversation of other people. Quit trying to finish their sentences. An even better sort of drill for you if you have been in the habit of hastening the other person's speech rhythms is to seek out a person who stutters and then deliberately remain tranquil.'

2 If you continue to need to talk unnecessarily, perhaps you ought to ask yourself the following questions: (1) Do I really have anything important to say? (2) Does anyone want to hear it? and (3) Is this the time to say it? If the answer to any one of these three questions is no, then remain quiet even if you find yourself biting your lips in frustration.

3 Try to control your obsessional time-directed life by making yourself aware of it and changing the established pattern of behaviour. For example, 'whenever you catch yourself speeding up your car in order to get through a yellow light at an intersection, penalize yourself by immediately turning to the right [or left] at the next corner. Circle the block and approach the same corner and signal light again. After such penalization you may find yourself racing a yellow light a second, but probably not a third time.' You can help yourself in nearly all aspects of your life, including social situations, by seeking out opportunities to control your Type A behaviour. 'Purposely, with a companion, frequent restaurants and theatres where you know there will be a period of waiting. If your companion is your wife, remember that you spend far longer periods of time alone with her in your own home without fidgeting. If you and your companion cannot find enough to say to each other as you wait in a restaurant or a theatre, then you had both better seek different companions.'

4 In order to put some of your Type A behaviour into perspective, carry out a number of exercises. Develop reflective periods in your self-created 'hectic program for life', creating opportunities to assess the causes of your hurry sickness. One of

the most important new habits to develop is a weekly review of the original causes of your present hurry sickness. Try to get to the source of your problems and current obsessions. Is your time-dominated behaviour really a need to feel important? Is it designed to avoid some activity or person? Is it really essential to the success of a particular goal? Friedman and Rosenman offer this advice: 'Never forget when confronted by any task to ask yourself the following questions: (1) will this matter have importance five years from now? and (2) must I do this right now, or do I have enough time to think about the best way to accomplish it?'

5 Try to understand that the majority of your work and social life does not really require 'immediate action', but instead requires a quality end product or a fulfilling relationship. 'Ask yourself, are good judgment and correct decisions best formulated under unhurried circumstances or under deadline pressures?'

6 As part of an effort to broaden yourself and lessen specific aspects of obsessional time-dictated behaviour, indulge in some outside activities: theatre, reading, sewing, and so on. Friedman and Rosenman recommend that patients 'for drill purposes, attempt to read books that demand not only your entire attention but also a certain amount of patience. We have repeatedly advised our Type A patients to attempt reading Proust's eight-volume novel *The Remembrance of Things Past* not because it is one of the great modern classics (which it is) but because the author needs several chapters to describe an event that most Type A subjects would have handled in a sentence or two.'

7 Try not to make unnecessary appointments or deadlines. 'Remember, the more unnecessary deadlines you make for yourself, the worse your "hurry sickness" becomes.'

8 Learn to protect your time and to say *No*. 'Try to never forget that if you fail to protect your allotment of time, no one else will. And the older you become, the more important this truth is.'

9 Take as many 'stress-free breathing spaces' during the course of an intensive working day as possible. 'Learn to interrupt long

or even short sessions of any type of activity that you know or suspect may induce tension and stress before it is finished. Such stress is particularly apt to arise in the course of writing long memos, reports or articles.' Taking the pressure off your stressful task – by reading the newspaper or taking a brief stretch – the kind of behaviour suggested here.

10 Try to create opportunities during the day or night when you can totally relax your body and mind.

Rosenman and Friedman also try to help the Type A person see how his behaviour affects his relationship with others:

1 Try to make yourself aware of the impact your behaviour has on other people. 'If you are overly hostile, certainly one of the most important drill measures you should adopt is that one in which you remind yourself of the fact that you are hostile.'

2 Try to reward people for their efforts. 'Begin to speak your thanks or appreciation to others when they have performed services for you. And do not do so, like so many hostile Type A subjects, with merely a grunt of thanks.' Such behaviour may seem unnatural at first, but it may help establish a different configuration of behaviours and extinguish the well-rehearsed hostile pattern. Try adopting a more relaxed and positive approach to people, greeting them regularly, taking time off to develop social relationships, and so on.

3 It is often the case that Type As blame other people for not meeting their ideals or find fault in others for their own failures or disappointments. 'Over and over again, we have listened to Type As rationalize their hostility as stemming from disappointment over the lack of ideals in their friends. We always have advised such sick people that they should cease trying to be "idealists" because they are in fact only looking for excuses to be disappointed and hence hostile towards others.'

While the above suggestions may seem unorthodox and in some cases extreme, they are a creative attempt to modify behaviour patterns which have been established for many years. A different orientation is to acknowledge the existence of your Type A behaviour and try to live comfortably with it. This requires an individual to become aware of his stress-related symptoms, such as stomach pains, and to take action to relieve them, such as taking time off work, or learning relaxation exercises, as will be discussed in the next section.

LEARNING TO RELAX

Life planning and changing long-lived behaviour patterns are major stress-reduction efforts that take time. You are not dealing with a simple problem and, as has been emphasized, there is usually not a single answer. But while you are investing the time and energy needed to sort out the stress factors in your life, there is some more immediate relief available to you – relaxation. A number of excellent books on the subject of stress control and relaxation have been written by stress management consultants who have used their ideas to help individuals and organizations with stress-related problems. We have already referred to three of these books – *Stress and the Manager: Making It Work For You*, by Karl Albrecht, *Organizational Stress and Preventive Management*, by James C. Quick and Jonathan D. Quick, and *Life After Stress*, by Martin Shaffer. Much of this section on relaxation and following sections on ways to control 'negative thought patterns' will be drawn from these excellent sources.

It is obvious that the body needs time to relax and recuperate from the effects of everyday stress. Some people can dissipate stress, while others 'bury it' deep within themselves. As Albrecht suggests, 'for these people life seems to be a series of crises. The chronically up-tight person seems to meet even a small problem as if it were a critical incident, as if somehow his survival were in jeopardy. A sudden call to come to the front office, a snag in a project schedule, a conflict with a co-worker, or a problem with a teenage son or daughter all take on the same apparent magnitude for the up-tight person. Such a person meets even the smallest problem situations with an unnecessarily intense reaction.'[8]

This kind of stress can reflect itself in a variety of personally damaging behaviours, such as excessive coffee or tea consumption, cigarette smoking, drug-taking and so forth. Most people believe, for example, that 'the coffee break' provides a useful stress-free breathing space, which it can do. It also, however, provides the individual with a further stimulant, as opposed to relaxant, which can actually adversely affect the biochemical balance in the body (that is, by depleting vitamins and minerals). In addition, the infusion of sugar (perhaps from doughnuts or sugar in coffee), which usually accompanies such coffee breaks, can lower the blood sugar level by stimulating insulin production and this can bring about a circular process with the body requiring even more intakes of sugar. This can lead in the short term to lower levels of body energy, and in the long term to potential weight gain.[9]

There are a whole range of activities we do during the course of each day which feel 'right' at the time, but which can have detrimental effects in the short or medium term. Shaffer's description of common 'misguided attempts to relax' can be found in Table 2.

Relaxation can combat some of these adverse reactions.[10] The evidence is mounting that relaxation techniques can provide the individual, through psychophysiological processes, with less damaging effects. The positive bodily outcomes of deep relaxation as a means of coping with peak arousal situations can be found in Table 3.

RELAXATION TECHNIQUES

There is a deep relaxation technique which you can use to try to achieve the relaxation response described above. It is a simple technique, which anyone can practise. If you feel somewhat tense about the thought of adding such a technique to your daily life, we suggest you make a commitment to practise relaxation on a daily basis for one month before deciding if you want to continue. Following this technique is a brief description of 'progressive relaxation', an alternative technique for which training or further study is required. The two techniques which follow this are shorter relaxation practices which you can use in addition to deep relaxation.

Table 2. Relaxing Activities

Pausing Activities	Purposes	Effects
Smoking cigarettes, tobaccos	Pick-me-up, pausing, arousal, social activity	Increased energy, nutrient drain, poor sleep, indigestion
Drinking coffee or tea (non-herbal)	Pausing, arousal, social activity	Energy boost, nutrient drain, poor sleep, indigestion
Drugs: cocaine, methadrine ('uppers')	Pick-me-up, arousal	Energy boost, nutrient drain, poor sleep, incoordination, hyperactivity
Drinking hard alcoholic beverages	Pausing, social activities, central nervous system depressant	Energy drain, digestive imbalance, potential brain impairment
Drinking wines	Pausing, social activities, central nervous system depressant, muscle relaxant	Energy drain
Drugs: marijuana and others	Pausing, social activities, muscle relaxant, vascular expansion	Energy drain, feeling 'wasted'
Eating sugary or highly refined foods	Pausing, arousal, pick-me-up, social activity	Poor nutrition, possible low blood sugar, possible indigestion

Source: Martin Shaffer, *Life After Stress* (Chicago: Contemporary Books, 1983).

Deep Relaxation Technique

For optimal effectiveness, deep relaxation is best done once or twice a day. It can help to assist your body in recovering from distress and prevent the build-up of tension, fatigue, and anxiety. Nita Catterton of the University of Virginia uses the following techniques:

Table 3. The Stress Response Versus the Relaxation Response

	Peak Arousal	Deep Relaxation
Adrenalin	More	Less
Respiration	Faster	Slower
Heart	Faster	Slower
Arteries	Constrict	Dilate
Blood pressure	Increase	Decrease
Metabolism	Faster	Slower
Muscle tension	Increase	Decrease
Stomach acid	More	Less
Blood sugar	More	Less
Insulin	More	Less
Cholesterol in blood	More	Less
Brain waves	Beta (i.e. less productive cognitive processes)	Alpha or theta (i.e. more creative cognitive processes)

Source: Nita Catterton, unpublished paper, University of Virginia.

1 Sit in a comfortable position. (Support your upper back, neck, and head.) A quiet place where you will not be interrupted is best.
2 Slowly draw in and exhale a deep breath. Check your shoulders for stiffness or tense position. Allow them to fall naturally in a relaxed position. Take in a second deep breath and close your eyes.
3 Complete a body check to locate any areas of tension and tightness. Take each area and relax the involved muscles. Visualize the tension releasing and slipping away as warmth and relaxation flow into the area. You might imagine yourself basking in the sun and feeling the sun warm your area of tension. (If you are having difficulty evaluating whether or not you are

relaxing a specific area try increasing the tension in the muscle and hold that tightness for a count of ten, then release.)

4 Starting with your feet, slowly work up through the body, relaxing muscle groups and areas of tightness and tension. Imagine warmth flowing into each area, muscles becoming heavy, and comforting relaxation replacing tightness or tension. Once you've progressed throughout your body, focus on your hands. (You can focus on any area of tension you'd like to work on.) Create a sentence that you can repeat to yourself emphasizing warmth, heaviness, and relaxation, such as, 'My hands are warm, heavy, and relaxed.'

5 Do not be discouraged if at first your mind tends to wander away to other thoughts. Once you are aware that you have wandered to other thoughts simply come back and focus again on the area you are relaxing. Try to notice how good it feels to have some quiet time to yourself and how comfortable it is to let go of any tightness or tension you may have.

6 Deep relaxation is most effective when practised for a length of twenty minutes. If you find that sitting still for that long is more stress-inducing than stress-reducing then start with a period of five or ten minutes and gradually build up to twenty minutes.

7 Always end your relaxation session with several deep breaths. Then, after slowly opening your eyes, maintain your relaxation position for a few minutes before resuming your next activity.

Make a commitment to practise deep relaxation on a daily basis for one month before determining if you want to continue with this stress-reduction technique.

Progressive Relaxation

Progressive Relaxation, as developed by Dr Edmund Jacobson, aims at reducing anxiety by emphasizing physical relaxation.[11] Jacobson combines both psychological awareness of stress factors with physiological manifestations and treatment. As it is currently taught, progressive relaxation consists of first tensing, then releasing all sixteen major skeletal muscle groups into which Jacobson has divided the body. As Quick and Quick describe it, 'The muscles are tensed for five to seven seconds and then relaxed for about thirty seconds. This process begins with the arms, progresses to the face, neck and throat, and then through the chest, abdomen, legs, and finally, the feet ... The whole process lasts thirty to sixty minutes. With experience, the subject learns to combine muscle groups into first seven and then four groups. It may take thirty hours or more to master the skill.'[12]

Two shorter relaxation exercises which take a maximum of ten minutes to practise can also be helpful. The following exercises, developed by Dr Cary McCarthy, are aimed at allowing an individual to evoke a feeling of peace and relaxation whenever desired.

Mental Relaxation (five to ten minutes)

1 Select a comfortable sitting or reclining position.
2 Close your eyes and think about a place that you have been before that represents your ideal place for physical and mental relaxation. (It should be a quiet environment, perhaps the seashore, the mountains, or even your own back garden. If you can't think of an ideal relaxation place, then create one in your mind.)
3 Now imagine that you are actually in your ideal relaxation place. Imagine that you are seeing all the colours, hearing the sounds, smelling the aromas. Just lie back, and enjoy your soothing, rejuvenating environment.
4 Feel the peacefulness, the calmness, and imagine your whole body and mind being renewed and refreshed.
5 After five to ten minutes, slowly open your eyes and stretch. You have the realization that you may instantly return to your relaxation place whenever you desire, and experience a peacefulness and calmness in body and mind.

Number Count Down (three to ten minutes)

1 Select a comfortable position.
2 Close your eyes, and breathe deeply and rhythmically several times.
3 Take another deep breath and, while exhaling, mentally visualize the number three (3). 3 is your symbol for complete body relaxation. (Relax any tension in your body, remembering the state of deep relaxation felt after the tensing muscle exercise.) Mentally repeat to yourself, '3, complete body relaxation'.

4 Take another deep breath, and while exhaling mentally visualize the number two (2). 2 is your symbol for complete brain and nervous system relaxation. (Any thoughts, fears, concerns, worries – let them all go. Relax all thought processes, feeling a sense of mental stillness and harmony.) Mentally repeat to yourself, '2, complete brain and nervous system relaxation'.

5 Take another deep breath, and while exhaling mentally visualize the number one (1). 1 is your symbol for complete 'oneness' within yourself, for complete attunement and harmony of mind and body. Mentally repeat to yourself, '1, oneness, mind-body harmony'.

6 In this deep state of mind-body relaxation, you are filled with calmness, peacefulness. You are at one with creative forces to bring about positive changes and benefits in your daily life and health. (At this time give yourself positive health suggestions you wish to hear. If there is a particular part of your body that needs healing, imagine that your own health energies are flowing to that part. Create a tingling sensation, and imagine the body area bathed in pure light energy, restoring and renewing every cell and tissue.)

7 When you are ready to continue with your daily activities, say to yourself, 'I have been in a deep, renewing state of mind-body relaxation. I will maintain the perfect attunement I have experienced, and will be in perfect health, feeling better than ever before. I will count from one to five, and at the count of five I will feel wide awake and in perfect health.'

8 Then begin counting, '1, 2, 3, 4, 5.' Open your eyes and say out loud (or repeat mentally with your eyes open), 'I am wide awake, in perfect health, feeling better than ever before.'

Meditation

Although a wide variety of meditation practices exist, Transcendental Meditation (TM) has been the most widely analysed in terms of its relief of stress. TM has been reported to help work adjustment through the reduction of tension. Researchers who have evaluated TM indicate it has lowered anxiety, increased job satisfaction and improved work performance.[13] TM has been shown to have long-term benefits as well, such as the reduction of high blood pressure levels. Although TM is increasingly being used in the treatment of hypertension and anxiety, there are those who contend it also has positive biochemical effects directly linked to stress-related illness.[14] Although such contentions will need confirmation through further research, it appears clear that TM can help the individual prepare his bodily processes for the pressures of everyday life. Approved TM instructors teach meditators to spend two daily twenty-minute sessions in a quiet, comfortable place silently repeating their mantra, the sound or word given to the trainee by the instructor. The trainee aims at developing a passive attitude and peaceful view of life.

The Relaxation Response

Based on their study of Transcendental Meditation, Herbert Benson and R. K. Peters devised a set of simple instructions designed to elicit the relaxation response described above.[15] The method involves sitting in a quiet, comfortable place, passively focusing on breathing and the word 'one'. Peters and Benson suggest the technique be practised for ten to twenty minutes once or twice a day, avoiding times immediately following meals. The instructions they give are as follows:

1 Sit quietly in a comfortable position.
2 Close your eyes.
3 Beginning at your feet and progressing up to your face, deeply relax your muscles. Keep them relaxed.
4 Breathe through your nose. Become aware of your breathing. As you breathe out, say the word 'one' silently to yourself. Continue the pattern; breathe in . . . out, one; in . . . out, one; and so on. Breathe easily and naturally.
5 Continue for ten to twenty minutes. You may open your eyes to check the time, but do not use an alarm. When you finish, sit quietly for several minutes, first with your eyes closed and later with your eyes opened. Do not stand up for a few minutes.
6 Do not worry about whether you are successful in achieving a deep level of relaxation. Maintain a passive attitude and permit relaxation to occur at its own pace. When distracting thoughts occur, try to ignore them by not dwelling on them and return to repeating 'one'. With practice, the

response should come with little effort. Practise the technique once or twice daily but not within two hours of any meal, since the digestive processes seem to interfere with eliciting the relaxation response.

Momentary Relaxation

While the relaxation exercises above require an investment in time, from a few minutes to twenty or more, once you have achieved deep relaxation you can also begin to draw upon your 'memory' of relaxation to achieve partial relaxation during the day. Taking a few deep, slow breaths can often bring on this feeling of relaxation. Albrecht states that the skill of momentary relaxation should come almost automatically once an individual has mastered a deep relaxation technique. With the following examples he describes the feeling of momentary relaxation:

The next time you find yourself about to deal with a challenging, stressful situation, simply pause for a few seconds, turn your attention to your body, and allow your whole body to relax as much as you can, keeping the situation in mind. You can easily learn to do this 'quickie' relaxation technique in a few seconds and without the slightest outward sign of what you are doing. Anyone looking at you would notice, at most, that you had become silent and that you seemed to be thinking about something for a few seconds. You need not even close your eyes to do this.

If you happen to have a few moments alone before entering the challenge situation, you can relax yourself somewhat more thoroughly. Sit down, if possible, get comfortable, and close your eyes. Use your built-in muscle memory to bring back the feeling of deep relaxation and hold it for about a full minute. Then open your eyes and, as you go about the task at hand, try to retain the feeling of calmness that came with the relaxation.[16]

Autogenic Training

Profound muscle relaxation is achievable through hypnosis, research has shown. Hypnosis is defined as an 'induced state of altered consciousness characterized by extreme relaxation and a heightened susceptibility to suggestion'.[17] A trained expert can induce a hypnotic trance by focusing an individual's attention on a mental or visual image, for example, by suggesting they think of something peaceful or repetitive. Many individuals can be trained to induce a hypnotic state in themselves through self-hypnosis. Self-hypnosis is best learned from an experienced practitioner, but can then be practised continually without further reinforcement.[18]

Quick and Quick describe autogenic training as a method of self-hypnosis which 'emphasizes the development of individual control over physiologic process through organ- and symptom-specific exercises'.[19] In a training process which usually takes between two and three months, the subject learns six standard training exercises aimed at inducing a general feeling of well-being and high coping ability. From this point, an individual goes on to learn 'organ-specific' exercises, which deal with particular psychophysiological dynamics, such as breathing, blood flow, and skin temperature. Once again, autogenic training succeeds best with the help of a trained therapist.[20]

PHYSICAL EXERCISE

Research is increasingly giving credence to the idea that exercise is good for the mind as well as the body. For example, Quick and Quick state that 'aerobically fit individuals' have been shown to have 'a better interplay between their activating, stress-response sympathetic nervous system and their relaxing, restorative parasympathetic nervous system. This suggests that fit individuals may be less psychologically reactive in stressful situations.'[21] Recent evidence suggests that vigorous exercise can lead to a biochemical change that improves one's psychological well-being as well as one's body conditioning.[22] Additional benefits of exercise include improved self-esteem, more restful sleep, a stronger and more attractive body, and reduction of anxiety and depression. Anyone considering starting to exercise should begin gradually. Also, many health organizations recommend that people above the age of thirty-five have their physician's approval before beginning a new exercise programme.

Aerobic exercise has received the most praise as a stress antidote. Through aerobic exercise, the individual's heart rate and respiration rate are sustained at a high level for twenty to thirty minutes. Jogging, brisk walking, aerobic dancing, and swimming are all aerobic exercises. According to Quick and Quick, 'aerobic exercise is the only form of exercise which can predictably achieve cardio-respiratory fitness'. Many new dieting theories maintain that exercising aerobically three to four times each week actually raises our bodies' metabolism rates, allowing us to burn more calories and lose weight.

Recreational sports such as squash and tennis can all be excellent ways of releasing tension and frustration, but they do not provide the aerobic benefits. Similarly, many people find that a favourite activity or hobby, such as gardening, sewing, listening to music, or soaking in a hot bath, can be tremendously helpful in releasing the build-up of tension. The key to such activities is that they can be done purely for the pleasure they bring. Although such traditional methods for relaxing have received little attention from researchers, many people know that engaging in a favourite activity can help repair the ravages of the day.

BIOFEEDBACK TRAINING

As we discussed in Chapter 1, the 'stress response' involves a complex interaction of hormones and nervous system responses. Through biofeedback, sensors attached to selected points on the body can measure a response such as a change in brain waves, blood pressure, heart rate, muscle tension or skin temperature. This response is measured through a blinking light or beeping tone. Most individuals learn fairly rapidly to get the light signal or tone to change in a desired way by reaching a certain level of deep relaxation or concentration. By paying attention to feelings and sensations experienced when the signal 'feeds back' information of tension or, conversely, relaxation, individuals can go on to regulate biological functions. Biofeedback training, used as a method for controlling adverse bodily reactions to stress, can be carried out in a lab setting, or by an individual with appropriate equipment and training.

EXPRESSING YOUR FEELINGS

In addition to taking advantage of the physical outlet provided by exercise and recreation, you may also find stress relief through talking or writing about your feelings. Venting frustration and anger to an understanding co-worker, friend or family member is one of the most common means of 'blowing off steam'.

Writing down your thoughts can also effectively reduce feelings of conflict or anger. Keeping a regular journal of your feelings or simply dashing off an angry letter that is either thrown away or later revised when emotions have cooled can be therapeutic.

SLEEP AND REST

Anyone who has experienced a sleep disturbance or insomnia can testify to the importance of sleep to overall functioning and mood. Sleep provides the body with a chance to recuperate and rebuild. As Shaffer describes it, 'the brain, which controls biological survival, needs rest to maintain its equilibrium . . . the brain, without adequate rest and sleep, cannot maintain the biochemical and electrical balances needed for effective functioning. Furthermore, when the brain is in such a state of disequilibrium, a person cannot cope effectively.'[23] Difficulty falling asleep, insomnia, and early morning awakening can all reflect depression or anxiety. Individuals who rely on alcohol to unwind and fall asleep in the evening may often find they awaken in the early morning when their bodies respond to an alcohol-induced adrenalin surge.[24]

Obviously, we all differ on the amount of sleep we need. Some people need few but continuous hours of sleep, while others need longer hours (say eight to ten hours). The ability to fall asleep quickly and sleep deeply appears to be improved by becoming relaxed before retiring (through a relaxation exercise or personal routine such as taking a warm bath); resolving, or consciously putting aside, emotional conflicts; avoiding overeating in the evening hours; and creating a sleeping environment that is comfortable in terms of light and temperature levels.

Resting during the daytime has also been shown to benefit bodies and minds. To be truly restful, a break must involve a real withdrawal from the day's activities. Often, even a brief change in scenery can be refreshing. Many people who work in a tight space find that lifting their eyes and gazing out of a window or at a pleasant painting or poster several times a day can be restful. Some research is available which suggests that daytime resting or breaks can moderate illness.[25]

STRESS AND GOOD NUTRITION

While much controversy exists about certain questions of diet and health, most stress researchers appear to agree about the value of eating to maintain level energy reserves through the day and to keep weight at a proper level.

The age-old adage, 'moderation in all things', seems to be sound advice today. Large amounts of sugar, processed foods, alcohol, and caffeine have been connected with poor overall health, irregular energy patterns and lowered resistance to illness and stress. As discussed above, many nutritionists argue that foods high in sugar cause a roller-coaster energy effect. Refined sugar is described as an 'empty food' which contributes nothing to the body and actually drains it of important nutrients.

Although diets abound, any sound weight-reducing effort will involve a revising of an individual's eating pattern to include fewer foods which are high in sugar and fat content, and more fresh foods which offer a good balance of protein and carbo-hydrates. An excellent discussion of eating for good health is offered in *Jane Brody's Good Food Book*, or Gail Duff's *Good Healthy Food*.[26]

COGNITIVE REAPPRAISAL – PERCEIVING THE STRESS FACTORS DIFFERENTLY

Relaxing, resting, exercising and eating well are all aimed at building your stress resiliency and lowering your reactivity to stressful events. The following section will examine ways of lowering your reactions to stressful events by managing your perceptions of daily events. As we discussed in earlier chapters, the way an individual perceives a situation dramatically affects the stress response experienced. For example, Type A individuals continually set off their stress responses by perceiving life as competitive and time-oriented. People who have an external locus of control perceive that they have little control over the situations which confront them daily. In contrast, the 'hardy personality' perceives he or she has a great deal of control of his life. In the last two cases, it is not so much the actual ability to cope with a situation as the individual's perception of his ability to cope that matters.

There are a range of techniques available to help cognitively reappraise many stressful situations. One such technique has been referred to by Quick and Quick as 'constructive self-talk'.[27]

They describe this as 'intermittent mental monologue' that most people conduct about the events they experience and their reactions to these events. This monologue or self-talk can range from being gently positive to harshly condemning. When someone engages in 'negative self-talk', they achieve nothing and just maintain the stress, dissipating their emotional energy. If you are involved in constructive self-talk, it can achieve more positive psychological results. Quick and Quick provide a range of examples of situations, 'mental monologues' and alternative strategy for constructive self-talk, which is shown here in Table 4.

Another technique one could use is what Albrecht refers to as 'quick recovery', that is, the ability to bounce back from upsetting experiences.[28] Learning to recover quickly takes little more than an awareness of how you actually do recover. As Albrecht describes it, 'once you begin to think about your emotional responses, you can recognize the process of returning to emotional equilibrium after a provocation has passed.' For example, if you find yourself drawn into a personal confrontation, you will very likely experience anger and a full-blown stress response. 'Your higher level mental processes will probably not be functioning very well,' Albrecht explains. 'However, at a certain point, your emotions will begin to subside and you will realize that you are angry. That is, you will experience your anger as an intellectual concept as well as a physical feeling.' Albrecht states that at this point, you have the option to continue and aggravate your angry feelings by 'rehashing the provocation, rejustifying your position, reopening a new attack on your adversaries, and becoming newly outraged by their unreasonable behaviour'. A quick recovery approach would suggest you stop this 'negative circular approach,

Table 4. Constructive Self-talk

Situation	Typical Mental Monologue	Constructive Self-talk Alternative
Driving to work on a day which you know will be full of appointments and potentially stressful meetings.	'Oh boy, what a day this will be!' 'It's going to be hell.' 'I'll never get it all done.' 'It'll be exhausting.'	'This looks like a busy day.' 'The day should be very productive.' 'I'll get a lot accomplished today.' 'I'll earn a good night's rest today.'
Anticipation of a seminar presentation or public address.	'What if I blow it?' 'Nobody will laugh at my opening joke.' 'What if they ask about . . .?' 'I hate talking to groups.'	'This ought to be a challenge.' 'I'll take a deep breath and relax.' 'They'll enjoy it.' 'Each presentation goes a bit better.'
Recovering from a heart attack.	'I almost died. I'll die soon.' 'I'll never be able to work again.' 'I'll never be able to play sports again.'	'I didn't die. I made it through.' 'The doctor says I'll be able to get back to work soon.' 'I can keep active and gradually get back to most of my old sports.'
Difficulty with a superior at work.	'I hate that person.' 'He makes me feel stupid.' 'We'll never get along.'	'I don't feel comfortable with him.' 'I let myself get on edge when he's around.' 'It will take some effort to get along.'
Flat tyre on a business trip.	'Damn this old car.' (Paces around car, looking at flat tyre.) 'I'll miss all my meetings.' 'It's hopeless.'	'Bad time for a flat.' (Begins to get tools out to start working.) 'I'll call and cancel Jenkins at the next phone. I should make the rest of the appointments.'

Source: J. C. Quick and J. D. Quick, *Organizational Stress and Preventive Management* (New York: McGraw-Hill, 1984), p. 221.

become more rational and less conscious of your need to 'win'.

The final two approaches which may prove helpful are what Quick and Quick refer to as 'thought stopping' and 'mental diversion'.[29] Thought-stopping means recognizing non-constructive thoughts, attitudes and behaviours and stopping them immediately – by visualizing, for example, a large STOP sign. Then one uses 'mental diversion' to divert the topic, issue, crisis to one that is manageable, until one has resources to cope with it. Or as Quick and Quick suggest, one way to stop a thought pattern is to divert yourself to a more positive topic.[30] For instance, once you have prepared yourself adequately for a coming event, such as a presentation or interview, obsessive worry can only drain your emotional resources. Diverting your thoughts to a more pleasant, restful subject can stop a negative thought pattern. It is often helpful to develop several topics as substitutes, such as memories of a favourite vacation, plans for a hobby project, or the words to a favourite song or poem.[31]

FINDING THE SUPPORT YOU NEED

In addition to all the self-help activities we described above, it is also important to find the social support you need. As discussed in Chapter 3, research has found social support a strong buffer against the stresses of work and life generally. A major source of support can be found among family members and friends. Also, the support and friendships developed at work can be extremely valuable.

Family Support: Coping with Family Stress

The changing roles in society, the increased presence of drugs, competitive tensions in the workplace and a myriad other factors combine to put the family unit under siege. What can the family do to help itself?

Firstly, before anything else, families must begin to communicate. Martin Shaffer has suggested different 'principles of clear communication' within a family unit to reduce the tensions and stress.[32] These principles attempt to clarify misunderstandings as they arise in the family unit. When there are tensions in a family, the 'pressure cooker' atmosphere frequently leads to false assumptions, misreadings of important verbal and non-verbal cues, and anticipatory behaviour that frustrate effective communication. Shaffer's format can provide the foundation for an atmosphere of greater trust and more open communication.[33] He advises:

1 Speak clearly.
2 Say what you mean with *complete* messages.
3 Be *specific* with regard to time, place, context, and reference.
4 Make non-verbal aspects of your message *congruent* with the verbal content of the message.
5 *Listen* carefully and actively, *without* mind-reading, assumptions, or judgements.
6 *Check out* and clarify that what you understand corresponds with what was intended.
7 *Complete transactions* until both parties have the same understanding of a message.

Once the communication systems are functioning within the family unit, alternative strategies or action plans can be developed to cope with conflicts. All members of the family must be involved. It might be useful in this context to adopt a strategy of semi-formalized family negotiation meetings, where issues of roles, boundaries, and conflicts are explored. This should not be a vague session where the individual members explode or are critical of the lack of family support, but a constructive, detailed and concise review of the conflict, time commitments, role confusion or whatever is undermining the cohesiveness of the family. This review of 'family accounts', as it were, should conclude by developing an action plan which distributes tasks among family members, or resolves some conflict, or in some other way follows through to resolution a significant issue for the family or one of its members. For example, if there are time commitment and role problems among family members, the following role negotiation strategy could be followed:

Step 1 Prepare a balance sheet of work and home commitments (listing details of hours spent, tasks undertaken, etc.).

Step 2 Call a formal family meeting to share concerns and discuss the detailed balance sheet.

Step 3 Re-negotiate various family commitments.

Step 4 Create mutual action plans for the next three months which are agreed by all family members.

Step 5 Review success, or otherwise, of action plans at the end of a three-month period.

Step 6 Develop new action plans based on experience of previous one. Continue the process until all parties are adequately satisfied with arrangements.

As described in Chapter 3, families can provide excellent support and education for their members. Open communication patterns, flexibility and the willingness to change can cement the relationships vital to this support.

Social Support at Work

In addition to strengthening family ties, individuals can seek support at work. One of the most important sources of social support is through the informal work group. The complicated set of relationships at work and their potential for conflict and ambiguity make it necessary for individuals to seek support from their peers. In this respect, there are a number of different approaches one can take. Firstly, those responsible for people within organizations should create the right atmosphere to encourage social support networks and to provide the most appropriate resources for stress management. Secondly, the individual can act to create these networks. Below are a number of steps an individual under stress may take to find social support at work:

1 Pick somebody at work you feel you can talk to; someone you don't feel threatened by and to whom you can trustfully reveal your feelings. Don't use people who, on reflection, you may be using on an unconscious level as a pawn in a game of organizational politics!

2 Approach this person and explain that you have a particular problem at work or outside work that you would like to discuss. Admit that you need help and that he or she would be the best

person to consult because you trust his or her opinion, like him or her as a person, and feel that he or she can usefully identify with your circumstances.

3 Try to maintain and build on this relationship, even at times of no crisis or problems.

4 Review, from time to time, the nature of the relationship, to see if it is still providing you with the emotional support you need to cope with the difficulties that arise. If the relationship is no longer constructive or the nature of your problems has changed (requiring a different peer counsellor), then seek another person for support.

It might be useful to have some method of selecting a peer counsellor. Fred Fiedler has provided a useful questionnaire, called the 'Most Preferred Co-worker Scale' (see p. 226), which might help in this regard, although it was not intended for this purpose. First think of the person you feel would help you the most in coping with your work stress. He or she may be someone you work with now or someone you knew in the past. Describe this person as he or she appears to you by placing an X above the appropriate number for each set of bi-polar adjectives. After you have completed this for all the items, if this person is not available try to think of someone currently in your workplace whom you feel you can trust.

This approach to social support at work may seem terribly contrived, but it is important for those of us in need of help to 'own up' to our difficulties and not to rely totally on the organization always to be there to resolve them. We must take personal initiatives to seek the kind of professional or 'peer' help that may be necessary, if we experience pressure at work we feel we can't adequately cope with ourselves.

COPING WITH REDUNDANCY

Individuals who have been made redundant need to be helped to cope with the experience at three different stages. Firstly, when they are initially made redundant, they will need social support to cope with the feelings of rejection and loss. This support must come from their spouse, family and very close friends. Secondly, for those who do not find immediate re-employment, additional support will be necessary to help them with the practical problems of financial planning, the job search, realistic assessment of their skills and abilities, retraining possibilities, and so on. Thirdly, for those who are among the growing band of long-term unemployed, they will need more substantive help in dealing with their depression, loss of self-worth, undermining of family role and the myriad other debilitating consequences of job loss. At the initial stage, the individuals have to come to terms with the need for personal and career counselling from trained professionals in the field. During this period, they must also find alternative activities to replace past paid work, in an effort to enhance their self-esteem, develop new skills and interests and to relieve the psychological stress within themselves and their family.

COPING WITH THE STRESS OF DUAL-CAREER FAMILIES

As trends begin to move away from Francine and Tim Hall's 'accommodator' marriage pattern to the dual-career family (see p. 130), we will find that the potential pressures in life will also increase at an exponential rate, depending on the type of pattern adopted. A number of people involved in this field have suggested coping strategies. Lotte Bailyn suggested that there are three strategies available to reduce the complexity of a marriage pattern based on the principle of equal sharing.[35] Firstly, she proposes the most obvious solution – the 'limitation of both partners' involvement in one or the other area' (that is domestic or work areas). By this she means that some form of role negotiation should take place whereby specific limitations for each member should be agreed. If, for example, neither member is prepared to accommodate the other's needs in terms of home commitments, it might be agreed to lessen family demands by having a smaller family or no family at all. In a work context it might mean negotiating more flexible working hours, or reducing time commitments, or sharing jobs. What is being done here, in effect, is limiting the demands from either or both areas of life in a way that allows both partners

Table 5. Most Preferred Co-worker Scale

	Very	Quite	Some-what	Slightly
Pleasant	8	7	6	5
Friendly	8	7	6	5
Rejecting	1	2	3	4
Helpful	8	7	6	5
Unenthusiastic	1	2	3	4
Tense	1	2	3	4
Distant	1	2	3	4
Cold	1	2	3	4
Co-operative	8	7	6	5
Supportive	8	7	6	5
Boring	1	2	3	4
Quarrelsome	1	2	3	4
Self-assured	8	7	6	5
Efficient	8	7	6	5
Gloomy	1	2	3	4
Open	8	7	6	5

Source: F. E. Fiedler, *A Theory of Leadership Effectiveness* (New York: McGraw-Hill, 1967)

Slightly	Some- what	Quite	Very	
				Unpleasant
4	3	2	1	
				Unfriendly
4	3	2	1	
				Accepting
5	6	7	8	
				Frustrating
4	3	2	1	
				Enthusiastic
5	6	7	8	
				Relaxed
5	6	7	8	
				Close
5	6	7	8	
				Warm
5	6	7	8	
				Uncooperative
4	3	2	1	
				Hostile
4	3	2	1	
				Interesting
5	6	7	8	
				Harmonious
5	6	7	8	
				Hesitant
4	3	2	1	
				Inefficient
4	3	2	1	
				Cheerful
5	6	7	8	
				Guarded
4	3	2	1	

an opportunity to cope in two worlds. Secondly, she suggests the notion of *recycling*, which is 'a shift in the staging of work and family events'. The main purpose of this is to organize events in such a way that work and home demands do not occur simultaneously or at least that the maximal demands do not overlap. This may mean that one member of the family has to delay a particular activity, be it an educational or occupational one, to a later period of the family's life cycle. It involves a great deal of long-term planning and the willingness to give up current interests and motivations until later stages in one's life. Bailyn continually indicates that the success of any of these strategies is highly contingent on the partners' ability and willingness to accommodate to each other and the family unit as a whole. And finally, she suggests *segmentation* as an approach to reduce complexity in dual-career marriages. This is defined as the process of 'strengthening the boundaries between family and work: by compartmentalizing each area so that one does not have to deal with family and work issues at the same time'. By making sure that one's world of work is dealt with during the 9 to 5 working day, it frees the individual to deal exclusively with family issues and problems at other times. This might extend to seeking out the type of employment and careers that will allow this. Once again the effort here is to plan activities so that they occur sequentially instead of simultaneously, thereby reducing the problems of overload or role conflict.

Bailyn's suggestions fit in nicely with what the Halls highlight as the three main stress agents among two-career couples: overload, conflict, and change.[36] One couple studied by the Halls described their overload as follows: 'When we're both under the gun at work, there's just no energy left for anything else. The apartment can go for a while, but what hurts is that neither of us has anything left at the end of the day for the other. At times like that there just isn't any support for anything or anyone. I don't know how people with kids handle it.' Or when there is a conflict of work and lifestyles: 'He is pulling back, putting more energy into relaxing. He wants me to play racquetball with him, but I come home late, have evening meetings, travel. I'm just getting my career launched, and he is cutting back on his. This has created a real problem for us – we're just coming from different directions. It's causing real strain in our relationship.' This will be a particular problem for those who adopt Bailyn's recycling strategy, which may inevitably lead to more synchronized workloads but also to differences in interest and direction at any given moment in time.

The Halls feel that the main answer to the problems experienced by two career couples is to develop a new career orientation and style, an approach they term the protean career (the term protean comes from the Greek mythological figure Proteus, who was able to change his form at will). They define *the protean career* as 'a process which the person, not the organization, is managing. It consists of all the person's varied experiences in education, training work in several organizations, changes in occupational field, etc. The protean career is not what happens to the person in any one organization. The protean person's own personal career choices and search for self-fulfilment are the unifying or integrative elements in his or her life. The criterion of success is internal (psychological success), not external. In short, the protean career is shaped more by the individual than by the organisation and may be redirected from time to time to meet the needs of the person.'[37] As the Halls emphasize, each person must take care of his or her own career rather than accept the inevitable organizational career paths and timetables. Once again the emphasis is on planning and self-determination.

CONCLUSION

If you have recognized a need to deal with stress in your life you have taken the first important step towards successfully dealing with the problem. This vital *recognition*, however important, must be matched equally with *determination* and *patience*. It is the determination to face truths about yourself and make necessary changes that will provide staying power when the going gets rough. In addition, you must have the patience to understand that change does not come about quickly; personal change and growth are both gradual processes.

NOTES

CHAPTER 1

1. L. E. Hinkle, 'The Concept of Stress in the Biological Social Sciences', *Stress Medicine and Man*, 1 (1973), 31–48.
2. H. Selye, 'The General Adaptation Syndrome and the Diseases of Adaptation', *Journal of Clinical Endocrinology*, 6 (1946), 117.
3. H. Basowitz, H. Persky, S. J. Karchin and R. R. Grinker, *Anxiety and Stress* (New York: McGraw Hill, 1955).
4. R. S. Lazarus, *Patterns of Adjustment* (New York: McGraw-Hill, 1976).
5. T. Cox, *Stress* (London: Macmillan, 1978).
6. T. Cummings and C. L. Cooper, 'A Cybernetic Framework for the Study of Occupational Stress', *Human Relations* vol. 32 (1979), 395–419.
7. A. Melhuish, *Executive Health* (London: Business Books, 1978).
8. K. Albrecht, *Stress and the Manager. Making It Work For You* (New Jersey: Prentice-Hall, 1979).
9. A. Melhuish, *op. cit.*
10. K. Albrecht, *op. cit.*
11. A. Melhuish, *op. cit.*
12. M. E. Carruthers, 'Risk Factor Control', paper presented to the conference entitled 'Stress of Air Traffic Control Officer', Manchester, April 1976.
13. B. H. Fox, 'Premorbid Psychological Factors as Related to Cancer Incidence', *Journal of Behavioural Medicine*, vol. 1, 1 (1978).
14. C. L. Cooper, R. Davies Cooper, E. B. Faragher, 'A Prospective Study of the Relationship Between Breast Cancer and Life Events. Type A Behaviour, Social Support and Coping Skills', *Stress Medicine*, vol. 2 (1986), 271–7.
15. J. C. Quick and J. D. Quick, *Organizational Stress and Preventive Management* (New York: McGraw-Hill, 1984).
16. J. C. Quick and J. D. Quick, *ibid.*
17. A. Melhuish, *op. cit.*
18. J. C. Quick and J. D. Quick, *op. cit.*

CHAPTER 2

1. Health Education Council, *Coronary Heart Disease Prevention – Plans for Action* (London: Pitman, 1984).

2. American Heart Association, *1986 Heart Facts* (Dallas, 1986).

3. C. L. Cooper, 'Job distress: Recent research and the emerging role of the clinical occupational psychologist', *Bulletin of the British Psychological Society*, 39 (1986), 325–31.

4. American Heart Association, *1986 Heart Facts* (Dallas, 1986).

5. American Heart Association, 1986, *ibid*.

6. American Heart Association, 1986, *ibid*.

7. L. Hawkins, M. White and L. Morris, 'Smoking, Stress and Nurses', *Nursing Mirror*, 13 October 1983.

8. American Heart Association, 1985, *ibid*.

9. A. Melhuish, *Executive Health* (London: Business Boots, 1978).

10. National Cancer Institute, *Cancer Rates and Risks*, US Department of Health and Human Services, 1985.

11. American Cancer Society, *Cancer Facts and Figures* (New York, 1986).

12. R. R. McCrea, P. T. Costa and R. Bosse, 'Anxiety, Extraversion and Smoking', *British Journal of Social and Clinical Psychology*, 17 (1978), 269–73.

13. P. Hingley and C. L. Cooper, *Stress and the Nurse Manager* (London: John Wiley, 1986).

14. American Cancer Society, *Cancer Facts and Figures* (New York, 1986).

15. *The President's Commission on Mental Health*, Stock no. 040-000-00390-8, US Government Printing Office (Washington, D.C., 1978).

16. T. J. Fischback, E. W. Dacey, J. P. Sestito and J. H. Green, *Occupational Characteristics of Disabled Workers*, 1975–6. Department of Health and Human Services, (NIOSH) Publication no. 86–106 (Washington, DC; 1986).

17. 'Top 200 Drugs of 1984: 2.1% Increase in Refill Pushes 1984 RxS 1.7% Ahead of 1983', *Pharmacy Times*, April 1985, 25–33.

18. C. Baum, D. L. Kennedy, D. E. Knapp and G. A. Faich, 'Prescription Drug Use in 1984': Paper presented at the American Public Health Association Annual Meeting (Washington, D.C., 1985).

19. A. Melhuish, *op. cit.*

20. 'Giving Mental Health its Research Due', *Science*, 232 (1986), 1065–1172.

21. B. K. Cypress, *Patterns of Ambulatory Care in International Medicine, the National Ambulatory Medical Care Survey*, United States,

January 1980–December 1981. *Vital and Health Statistics*, series 13, no. 80, DHHS Pub. no. (PHS) (Washington, D.C., 1984), 84–1741.

22. A. Melhuish, *op. cit.*

23. M. D. Good, B. J. Good and A. J. Massi, 'Patient Requests in Primary Health Care Settings: Development and Validation of a Research Instrument, *Journal of Behavioral Medicine*, 6 (1983), 151–68.

24. J. H. Nickalson, M. S. Donaldson and J. E. Oh, 'HMO Members and Clinicians Rank Health Education Needs', *Public Health Reports*, 98 (1983), 22–226.

25. *National Strategy on Prevention of Work-related Psychological Disorders* (Cincinnati: NIOSH, October 1986).

26. School for Advanced Urban Studies (SAUS), *Alcohol Education Programme Regional Profile* (Bristol: University of Bristol, 1985).

27. H. Selye, *Stress in Health and Disease* (London: Butterworth, 1976).

28. P. Hingley and C. L. Cooper, *op. cit.*

29. SAUS, *op. cit.*

30. National Institute on Alcohol Abuse and Alcoholism, *Alcohol World Health and Research*, vol. 9: No. 2 (1984/5).

31. S. Sloan and C. L. Cooper, *Pilots Under Stress* (London: Routledge and Kegan Paul, 1986).

32. V. Sutherland and C. L. Cooper, *Man and Accidents Offshore* (London: Lloyds of London Press, 1986).

33. V. D. Lachman, *Stress Management: a Manual for Nurses* (New York: Grune and Stratton, 1983).

34. Department of Health and Social Security, *Drinking Sensibly* (London: HMSO) 1981.

35. T. M. Rohan, 'Pushers on the Payroll: a Nightmare for Management', *Industry Week*, 212 (1982), 52.

36. T. M. Rohan, *ibid.*

37. R. P. Quinn and G. L. Staines, *The 1977 Quality of Employment Survey: Descriptive Statistics, with Comparison Data From the 1969–70 and the 1972–3 Survey* (University of Michigan: Ann Arbor, 1979).

38. E. Bolinder and B. Ohlstrom, *Stress pa Svenska Arbetsplatser: en Enkatstudie Bland LO-Medlemmasrna*, Prima/LO, Lund, 1971.

39. C. Maslach and A. Pines, 'Burnout: the Loss of Human Caring' in *Experiencing Social Psychology*, edited by C. Maslach (New York: Random House, 1979).

40. M. J. Colligan, M. J. Smith and J. J. Hurrell, 'Occupational Incidence Rates of Mental Health Disorders', *Journal of Human Stress*, 3 (1977), 34–9.

41. A. Melhuish, *op. cit.*
42. Confederation of British Industries, *Absenteeism: an Analysis of the Problem* (London: Confederation of British Industry, 1970).
43. P. Hingley and C. L. Cooper, *op. cit.*
44. J. C. Quick and J. D. Quick, *Organizational Stress and Preventive Management*.
45. K. Albrecht, *Stress and the Manager: Making it Work For You* (New Jersey: Prentice-Hall, 1979).
46. J. S. Lubin, 'On-the-job Stress Leads Many Workers to File, and Win, Compensation Awards', *Wall Street Journal*, 17 September 1980.
47. J. M. Ivancevich, M. T. Matteson and Edward P. Richards, 'Who's Liable For Stress on the Job?', *Harvard Business Review*, March–April 1985.
48. National Council on Compensation Insurance, *Emotional Stress in the Workplace – New Legal Rights in the Eighties* (NCCI: New York, 1985).
49. J. C. Quick and J. D. Quick, *op. cit.*

CHAPTER 3

1. M. Friedman, *Pathogenesis of Coronary Artery Disease* (New York: McGraw-Hill, 1969).
2. R. H. Rosenman, M. Friedman and R. Straus, 'A Predictive Study of CHD, *Journal of the American Medical Association*, 189 (1964), 15–22.
3. D. Jenkins, 'Psychologic and Social Precursors of Coronary Disease', *New England Journal of Medicine* 284, 6 (1971), 307–17.
4. R. H. Rosenman, M. Friedman and R. Straus, *op. cit.* Also by the same authors, 'CHD in the Western Collaborative Group Study', *Journal of the American Medical Association*, 195 (1966), 86–92.
5. R. D. Caplan, S. Cobb, J. R. P. French, R. Van Harrison and S. R. Pinneau, *Job Demands and Worker Health: Main Effects and Occupational Differences*, NIOSH Research Report (1975).
6. J. H. Howard, D. A. Cunningham and P. A. Rednitzer, 'Health Patterns Association with Type A Behaviour, A Managerial Population', *Journal of Human Stress*, vol. 2 (1976).
7. C. Mettlin, 'Occupational Careers and the Prevention of Coronary Prone Behaviour', *Social Science and Medicine*, 10 (1976), 367–72.
8. M. A. Chesney and R. H. Rosenman, 'Type A Behaviour in the Work Setting' in C. L. Cooper and R. Payne (eds.), *Current Concerns in Occupational Stress* (Chichester: John Wiley, 1980).

9. M. D. Friedman and R. H. Rosenman, *Type A Behavior and Your Heart* (New York: Knopf, 1974).

10. R. W. Bortner, 'A Short Rating Scale as a Potential Measure of Pattern A Behavior', *Journal of Chronic Diseases*, 22 (1969), 87–91.

11. Suzanne Kobasa, 'Conceptualization and Measurement of Personality in Job Stress Research', NIOSH Symposium, *Measures of Job Stress Workshop*, New Orleans, 21–3 October 1985.

12. Suzanne Kobasa, 'Stressful Life Events, Personality, Health: an Enquiry into Hardiness', *Journal of Personality and Social Psychology*, vol. 37 (1979).

13. J. B. Rotter, 'Generalised Expectations for Internal Versus External Control of Reinforcement', *Psychology Monograph*, 80 (1966).

14. *Ibid.*

15. D. Peck and D. Whitlow, *Approaches to Personality Theory* (London: Methuen, 1975).

16. J. H. Greer, G. C. Davison and R. I. Crutchel, 'Reduction of Stress in Humans Through Nonveridical Perceived Control of Adverse Stimulation', *Journal of Personality and Social Psychology*, 16 (1970), 731–8. Also D. Glass, J. E. Singer and L. N. Friedman, 'Psychic Cost of Adaption to an Environment Stressor', *Journal of Personality and Social Psychology*, 12, 200–210.

17. R. S. Lazarus, 'Cognitive and Personality Factors Underlying Threat and Coping' in M. H. Appley and R. Turnbull (eds.), *Psychological Stress* (New York: Appleton, 1967).

18. C. L. Cooper, *Stress Check* (New Jersey: Prentice-Hall, 1980).

19. C. L. Cooper, R. Davies Cooper and E. B. Faragher, 'A Prospective Study of the Relationship Between Breast Cancer and Life Events. Type A Behaviour, Social Support and Coping Skills', *Stress Medicine*, vol. 2 (1986), 271–7.

20. T. H. Holmes and M. Masuda, 'Life Change and Illness Susceptibility', *Separation and Depression*, AAAS (1973), 161–86.

21. C. L. Cooper (1980), op. cit.

22. A. R. Wyler, T. H. Holmes and M. Masuda, 'Magnitude of Life Events and Seriousness of Illness', *Psychosomatic Medicine*, 33 (1971) 115–22.

23. J. C. Quick and J. D. Quick, *Organizational Stress and Preventive Management*.

24. A. McLean, *Work Stress* (Boston: Addison-Wesley, 1979).

25. M. Davidson and C. L. Cooper, *Stress and the Woman Manager* (New York: St Martin's Press, 1983).

26. H. G. Wolff, *Stress and Disease* (Illinois: Charles C. Thomas, 1953).

27. M. G. Marmot and others, 'Epidemiologic Studies of Coronary Heart Disease and Stroke in Japanese Men Living in Japan, Hawaii and California', *American Journal of Epidemiology*, 102, 6 (1975), 514–25.

28. S. Gore, 'The Effects of Social Supports in Moderating the Health Consequences of Unemployment', *Journal of Health and Social Behaviour*, 19 (1978), 15–165.

29. R J. Burk, J. Frith and C. McGratten, 'Husband–Wife Compatibility and the Management of Stress', *Journal of Social Psychology*, 94 (1974), 243–52.

30. L. Eitinger and A. Strom, 'Mortality and Morbidity After Excessive Stress: a Follow-up Investigation of Norwegian Concentration Camp Survivors', *Humanities* (1973).

31. G. Caplan, 'The Family as a Support System' in G. Caplan and M. Killilea (eds.), *Support Systems and Mutual Help* (New York: Grune and Stratton, 1967).

32. L. Coch and J. R. P. French, 'Overcoming Resistance to Change', *Human Relations*, 1 (1948), 512–32.

33. J. R. P. French and R. D. Caplan, 'Organizational Stress and Individual Strain' in A. J. Marrow (ed.), *The Failure of Success* (New York: AMACOM, 1972), 30–60.

34. B. L. Margolis, W. H. Kroes and R. P. Quinn, 'Job Stress: an Unlisted Occupational Hazard', *Journal of Occupational Medicine*, 16 (10) (1974), 654–61.

35. J. M. La Rocco and A. P. Jones., 'Coworker and Leader Support as Moderators of Stress. Strain Relationships in Work Situations', *Journal of Applied Psychology*, 63, S (1978), 629–34.

36. E. Q. Wilson, *Sociobiology* (Cambridge, Mass.: Harvard University Press, 1975).

CHAPTER 4

1. S. Sloan and C. Cooper, *Pilots Under Stress* (London: Routledge and Kegan Paul, 1986).

2. M. Smith, M. Colligan, R. Horning and J. Hurrell, *Occupational Comparison of Stress-Related Disease Incidence* (Cincinnati: National Institute for Occupational Safety and Health, March, 1978).

3. A. McLean, *Work Stress* (Boston: Addison-Wesley, 1979).

4. C. L. Cooper, *Stress Check* (New Jersey: Prentice-Hall, 1981).

5. A. Kornhauser, *Mental Health of the Industrial Worker* (New York: John Wiley, 1965).

6. M. Kelly and C. L. Cooper, 'Stress Among Blue Collar Workers', *Employee Relations*, 3 (1981), 6–9.

7. D. Hay and D. Oken, 'The Psychological Stresses of Intensive Care Nursing', *Psychosomatic Medicine*, 34 (1972), 109–118.

8. P. Hingley and C. L. Cooper, *Stress and the Nurse Manager* (Chichester: John Wiley, 1986).

9. J. M. Ivancevich and M. T. Matteson, *Stress and Work* (Illinois: Scott, Foresman and Company, 1980).

10. *Ibid.*

11. S. Cobb and R. H. Rose, 'Hypertension, Peptic Ulcer and Diabetes in Air Traffic Controllers', *Journal of the Australian Medical Association*, 224 (1973), 489–92.

12. V. Sutherland and C. L. Cooper., *Man and Offshore Accidents* (London: Lloyds, 1987).

13. D. Tasto, M. Colligan, E. Skjei and S. Polly, *Health Consequences of Shiftwork*, NIOSH, US Government Printing Office (Washington, D.C., 1978).

14. L. Breslow, P. Buell, 'Mortality from Coronary Heart Disease and Physical Activity of Work in California', *Journal of Chronic Diseases*, 11, 615–25.

15. H. I. Russek, and B. L. Zohman, 'Relative Significance of Heredity, Diet and Occupational Stress in CHD of Young Adults', *American Journal of Medical Sciences*, 235, 266–75.

16. C. L. Cooper, 'Executive Stress: a Ten Country Comparison', *Human Resource Management*, 23 (1974), 395–407.

17. J. R. P. French and R. D. Caplan, 'Organizational Stress and Individual Strain', in A. Marrow (ed.), *The Failure of Success*.

18. *Ibid.*

19. T. Cox, 'Repetitive Work', in C. L. Cooper and R. Payne (eds.), *Current Concerns in Occupational Stress* (Chichester: John Wiley, 1980).

20. Joseph Heller, *Something Happened!* (New York: Ballantine Books, 1975).

21. L. J. Warshaw, *Managing Stress* (Reading, Mass.: Addison-Wesley, 1979).

22. J. M. Ivancevich and T. Matteson, *op. cit.*

23. J. C. Quick and J. D. Quick, *Organizational Stress and Preventive Management* (New York: McGraw-Hill, 1984).

24. P. Hingley and C. L. Cooper, *op. cit.*

25. J. C. Quick and J. D. Quick, *op. cit.*

26. J. M. Ivancevich and M. T. Matteson, *op. cit.*

27. C. L. Cooper, M. Mallinger and R. Kahn, 'Identifying Sources of Occupational Stress Among Dentists', *Journal of Occupational Psychology*, 51 (1978), 227–34.

28. P. Warr and T. Wall, *Work and Well-Being* (Harmondsworth: Penguin, 1975), 197–205.
29. W. Wardwell, I. M. Hyman and C. B. Bahnson, 'Stress and Coronary Disease in Three Field Studies', *Journal of Chronic Disease*, 17 (1964), 73–4.
30. A. Pincherle, 'Fitness for Work', *Proceedings of the Royal Society of Medicine*, 65 (1972), 321–4.
31. J. M. Ivancevich and M. T. Matteson, *op. cit.*
32. W. H. Kroes, *Society's Victim – the Policeman* (Illinois: C. C. Thomas, 1980).
33. J. H. Crump, C. L. Cooper and J. M. Smith, 'Investigating Occupational Stress: a Methodological Approach', *Journal of Occupational Psychology*, 1 (1980), 191–202.
34. H. Selye, *Stress Without Distress* (Philadelphia: J. B. Lippincott, 1974).
35. R. S. Lazarus, *Psychological Stress and Coping Process* (New York: McGraw-Hill, 1966).
36. J. R. P. French and R. D. Caplan, *op. cit.*
37. V. Buck, *Working Under Pressure* (London: Staples Press, 1972).
38. D. Gower and K. Legge, 'Stress and External Relationships – the Hidden Contract' in Gower and Legge (eds.), *Managerial Stress* (Epping: Gower Press, 1975).
39. C. L. Cooper and J. Marshall, *Understanding Executive Stress* (London: Macmillan, 1978).
40. J. R. P. French and R. D. Caplan in A. J. Marrow (ed.), *The Failure of Success* (New York: AMACOM, 1972), 31–66.
41. J. C. Quick and J. D. Quick, *op. cit.*
42. C. L. Cooper and R. Davies-Cooper, 'Occupational Stress Among International Interpreters', *Journal of Occupational Medicine*, 25 (1983), 889–95.
43. H. Levinson, 'The Abrasive Personality', *Harvard Business Review*, 56, May 1978.
44. K. Lewin, B. Lippitt and R. K. White, 'Patterns of Aggressive Behaviour in Experimentally Created Social Climates', *Journal of Social Psychology*, 10, 271–99.
45. J. C. Quick and J. D. Quick, *op. cit.*
46. J. M. Ivancevich and M. T. Matteson, *op. cit.* See also B. Blau, 'Understanding Mid-Career Stress', *Management Review*, 67 (1978), 57–62.
47. A. McGoldrick and C. L. Cooper, 'Stress at the Decline of One's Career: the Act of Retirement', in Terry A. Beerr and Rabis Bhagat (eds.) (New York: John Wiley, 1985).

48. E. R. Burgess (ed.), *Aging in Western Society: a Comparative Survey* (University of Chicago Press, 1960).

49. L. Coch and J. R. P. French, 'Overcoming Resistance to Change', *Human Relations*, 1 (1948), 512–32.

50. B. Margolis, W. Kroes and R. Quinn, 'Job Stress: an Unlisted Occupational Hazard', *Journal of Occupational Medicine*, 16, 10 (1974), 654–61.

51. R. L. Kahn, D. M. Wolfe, R. P. Quin, J. R. Snoek and R. N. Rosenthal, *Organizational Stress* (New York: John Wiley, 1964).

52. C. L. Cooper, 'Executive Stress: a Ten Country Comparison', *Human Resource Management*, 23 (1984), 395–407.

53. C. L. Cooper and M. Davidson, *High Pressure* (London: Fontana, 1982).

54. L. Larwood and M. Wood, *Women in Management* (London: Lexington Books, 1979).

55. K. Horner, *Femininity and Successful Achievement: a Basic Inconsistency. Feminine Personality and Conflict* (California: Brooks/Cole, 1970).

56. D. C. McClelland, *Power – The Inner Experience* (New York: Irvington, 1975).

57. S. G. Haynes, and M. Feinleib, 'Women, Work and Coronary Heart Disease: Prospective Findings from the Framingham Heart Study', *American Journal of Public Health*, 70 (1980), 133–41.

58. C. L. Cooper, S. Sloan and S. Williams, *Occupational Stress Indicator* (Windsor: NFER-Nelson, 1987).

CHAPTER 5

1. A. Toffler, *Future Shock* (London: Pan, 1970).

2. J. M. Ivancevich and M. T. Matteson, *Stress and Work* (Illinois: Scott, Foresman and Company, 1980).

3. See J. W. Mills, *Coping with Stress: a Guide to Living* (New York: John Wiley, 1982).

4. C. L. Cooper, *Executive Families Under Stress* (New Jersey: Prentice-Hall, 1982).

5. M. Henning and A. Jardim, *The Managerial Woman* (London: Pan, 1979).

6. C. Handy, 'The Family: Help or Hindrance', in C. L. Cooper and R. Payne (eds.), *Stress at Work* (London: John Wiley, 1978), 107–23.

7. F. S. Hall and D. T. Hall, *The Two-career Couple* (Mass.: Addison-Wesley, 1980).

8. J. R. Renshaw, 'He Can't Even Manage His Own Family', *Wharton Magazine* (Winter 1977), 42–7.
9. T. Parsons, *Essays in Sociological Theory* (Illinois: Free Press, 1954).
10. R. Pahl, 'Review of Dual-Career Families', *New Society*, vol. 19, 1971.
11. R. Rapoport and R. N. Rapoport, *Dual-Career Families* (Harmondsworth: Penguin, 1971).
12. A. C. Bebbington, 'The Function of Stress in the Establishment of the Dual-career Family', *Journal of Marriage and the Family* (1973), 530–37.
13. F. S. Hall and D. T. Hall, *op. cit.*
14. S. Orden and B. Orden, 'Working Wives and Marriage Happiness', *American Journal of Sociology*, vol. 74 (1969), 392–407.
15. R. O. Blood, 'Long-range Causes and Consequences of the Employment of Married Women', *Journal of Marriage and the Family* (1965), 43–7.
16. R. O. Blood and R. L. Hamblin, 'The Effect of the Wife's Employment on the Family Power Structure', *Social Forces* (1959), 347–52.
17. L. M. Cohen, 'Women's Entry to the Professions in Columbia: Selected Characteristics', *Journal of Marriage and the Family*, vol. 19 (1973).
18. A. E. Siegel, *et al.*, 'Dependence and Independence in Children' in L. Hoffman and I. Nye (eds), *The Employed Mother in America* (New York: Rand, 1963).
19. L. W. Hoffman, 'Mother's employment of work and effects on the child', in Hoffman and Nye (eds.), *ibid.*
20. N. Y. Zajur and E. Ocio, 'Leisure, Work and Women', *Revista Española de la Opinion Publica* (1972), 251–97.
21. J. E. Tropman, 'The Married Professional Social Worker', *Journal of Marriage and the Family* (1968), 661–5.
22. J. M. Ivancevich and M. T. Matteson, *op. cit.*
23. J. Marshall and C. L. Cooper, *Executive Under Pressure* (London: Macmillan, 1979).
24. J. M. Ivancevich and M. T. Matteson, *op. cit.*
25. *Ibid.*
26. A. Pettigrew, 'Managing Under Stress', *Management Today*, April 1972.
27. D. Fryer and R. Payne, 'Being Unemployed', in C. L. Cooper and I. Robertson (eds.), *International Review of Industrial and Organizational Psychology* (Chichester: John Wiley, 1986).
28. J. Hayes and P. Nutman, *Understanding the Unemployed*, (London: Tavistock Publ., 1981).

CHAPTER 6

1. R. D. Alberti and M. L. Emmons, *Your Perfect Right: a Guide to Assertive Behaviour* (New York: Impact, 1970).
2. S. Langrish, 'Assertiveness Training', in C. L. Cooper (ed.), *Improving Interpersonal Relations* (Epping: Gowen Press, 1981).
3. M. D. Galassi and J. P. Galassi, *Assert Yourself: How to Be Your Own Person* (New York: Human Sciences Press, 1977).
4. M. Davidson and C. L. Cooper, *Stress and the Woman Manager* (Oxford: Blackwell, 1983).
5. M. Henning and A. Jardim, *The Managerial Woman* (London: Pan Books, 1979).
6. C. Handy, *Understanding Organizations* (Harmondsworth: Penguin, 1976).
7. E. Flamholtz, 'Should Your Organization Attempt to Value its Human Resources', *California Management Review*, vol. 10, 1971.
8. C. L. Cooper, *Executive Families Under Stress* (New Jersey: Prentice-Hall, 1982).
9. J. Bensahel, 'Why Competition May Not Always Be Healthy', *International Management*, October 1978, 23–5.
10. C. L. Cooper, *op. cit.*
11. L. W. Foster, *et al.*, 'The Effects and Promises of the Shortened Work Week', *Academy of Management Proceedings*, August 1979.
12. M. P. Fogarty, R. Rapoport and R. N. Rapoport, *Sex, Career and Family* (Beverly Hills: Sage, 1971).
13. S. Ekberg-Jordan, 'Preparing for the Future', *Atlanta Economic Review*, March 1976, 47–9.
14. C. Handy, 'The Shape of Organizations to Come', *Personnel Management*, June 1979, 24–6.
15. E. De Bono, *Opportunities* (London: Associated Book Publishers, 1978).
16. C. L. Cooper and M. Davidson, *High Pressure* (London: Fontana, 1982).
17. T. Lidz, *The Person: Development Through the Life Cycle* (New York: Basic Books, 1968).
18. A. Mant, *The Rise and Fall of the British Manager* (London: Pan Books, 1977).
19. A. Kornhauser, *The Mental Health of the Industrial Worker* (New York: John Wiley, 1965).

CHAPTER 7

1. W. W. Dyer, *Your Erroneous Zones* (New York: Avon Books, 1976).
2. M. Shaffer, *Life After Stress* (Chicago: Contemporary Books, 1983).
3. K. Albrecht, *Stress and the Manager: Making It Work For You* (New Jersey: Prentice-Hall, 1979).
4. J. W. Pfeiffer and J. E. Jones, *Structural Experiences for Human Relations Training* (Iowa City: University Associates Press, 1970).
5. A. Lakein, *How to Get Control of Your Time and Your Life* (New York: Wyden, 1973).
6. M. Shaffer, *op. cit.*
7. M. D. Friedman and R. H. Rosenman, *Type A Behavior and Your Heart* (New York: Knopf, 1974).
8. K. Albrecht, *op. cit.*
9. M. Shaffer, *op. cit.*
10. S. Kasl and C. L. Cooper, *Stress and Health* (Chichester: John Wiley, 1987).
11. E. Jacobson, *Progressive Relaxation* (Chicago: University of Chicago Press, 1958).
12. J. C. Quick and J. D. Quick, *Organizational Stress and Preventive Management* (New York: McGraw-Hill, 1984).
13. D. J. Kuna, 'Meditation and Work', *Vocation Guidance Quarterly*, 23 (4) (1975).
14. H. Benson, *et al.*, 'Decreased Systolic Blood Pressure in Hypertensive Subjects Who Practiced Meditation', *Journal of Clinical Investigation*, 52 (1973).
15. R. K. Peters and H. Benson, 'Time Out For Tension', *Harvard Business Review*, February 1979.
16. K. Albrecht, *op. cit.*
17. B. S. Sachs, 'Hypnosis in Psychiatry and Psychosomatic Medicine', *Psychosomatics*, vol. 23 (1982), 523–5.
18. J. C. Quick and J. D. Quick, *op. cit.*
19. J. C. Quick and J. D. Quick, *ibid.*
20. B. Jencks, *Exercise Manual for Autogenic Training* (Illinois: American Society for Clinical Hypnosis, 1979).
21. J. C. Quick and J. D. Quick, *op. cit.*
22. S. R. Gambert, 'Exercise and the Endogenous Opioids', *New England Journal of Medicine*, 305 (1981), quoted in Quick and Quick, *op. cit.*
23. M. Shaffer, *op. cit.*
24. J. C. Quick and J. D. Quick, *op. cit.*
25. M. Shaffer, *op. cit.*

26. Jane Brody, *Jane Brody's Good Food Book* (New York: Norton and Company, 1985); Gail Duff, *Good Healthy Food* (Harmondsworth: Penguin, 1985).

27. J. C. Quick and J. D. Quick, *op. cit.*

28. K. Albrecht, *op. cit.*

29. J. C. Quick and J. D. Quick, *op. cit.*

30. J. C. Quick and J. D. Quick, *ibid.*

31. K. Albrecht, *op. cit.*

32. M. Shaffer, *op. cit.*

33. M. Shaffer, *ibid.*

34. F. E. Fiedler, *A Theory of Leadership Effectiveness* (New York: McGraw-Hill, 1967).

35. L. Bailyn, 'Career and Family Orientations of Husbands and Wives in Relation to Marital Happiness', *Human Relations*, 23 (1970), 97–113.

36. F. S. Hall and D. T. Hall, 'Stress and the Two Career Couple', in C. L. Cooper and R. Payne (eds.), *Current Concerns in Occupational Stress* (Chichester: John Wiley, 1980), 243–65.

37. F. S. Hall and D. T. Hall, *ibid.*

INDEX

READ MORE IN PENGUIN

In every corner of the world, on every subject under the sun, Penguin represents quality and variety – the very best in publishing today.

For complete information about books available from Penguin – including Puffins, Penguin Classics and Arkana – and how to order them, write to us at the appropriate address below. Please note that for copyright reasons the selection of books varies from country to country.

In the United Kingdom: Please write to *Dept. EP, Penguin Books Ltd, Bath Road, Harmondsworth, West Drayton, Middlesex UB7 0DA*

In the United States: Please write to *Consumer Sales, Penguin USA, P.O. Box 999, Dept. 17109, Bergenfield, New Jersey 07621-0120*. VISA and MasterCard holders call 1-800-253-6476 to order Penguin titles

In Canada: Please write to *Penguin Books Canada Ltd, 10 Alcorn Avenue, Suite 300, Toronto, Ontario M4V 3B2*

In Australia: Please write to *Penguin Books Australia Ltd, P.O. Box 257, Ringwood, Victoria 3134*

In New Zealand: Please write to *Penguin Books (NZ) Ltd, Private Bag 102902, North Shore Mail Centre, Auckland 10*

In India: Please write to *Penguin Books India Pvt Ltd, 706 Eros Apartments, 56 Nehru Place, New Delhi 110 019*

In the Netherlands: Please write to *Penguin Books Netherlands bv, Postbus 3507, NL-1001 AH Amsterdam*

In Germany: Please write to *Penguin Books Deutschland GmbH, Metzlerstrasse 26, 60594 Frankfurt am Main*

In Spain: Please write to *Penguin Books S. A., Bravo Murillo 19, 1° B, 28015 Madrid*

In Italy: Please write to *Penguin Italia s.r.l., Via Felice Casati 20, I–20124 Milano*

In France: Please write to *Penguin France S. A., 17 rue Lejeune, F–31000 Toulouse*

In Japan: Please write to *Penguin Books Japan, Ishikiribashi Building, 2–5–4, Suido, Bunkyo-ku, Tokyo 112*

In Greece: Please write to *Penguin Hellas Ltd, Dimocritou 3, GR–106 71 Athens*

In South Africa: Please write to *Longman Penguin Southern Africa (Pty) Ltd, Private Bag X08, Bertsham 2013*

READ MORE IN PENGUIN

A SELECTION OF HEALTH BOOKS

The Kind Food Guide   Audrey Eyton

Audrey Eyton's all-time bestselling *The F-Plan Diet* turned the nation on to fibre-rich food. Now, as the tide turns against factory farming, she provides the guide destined to bring in a new era of eating.

Baby and Child   Penelope Leach

This comprehensive, authoritative and practical handbook is an essential guide, with sections on every stage of the first five years of life.

Woman's Experience of Sex   Sheila Kitzinger

Fully illustrated with photographs and line drawings, this book explores the riches of women's sexuality at every stage of life. 'A book which any mother could confidently pass on to her daughter – and her partner too' – *Sunday Times*

The Effective Way to Stop Drinking   Beauchamp Colclough

Beauchamp Colclough is an international authority on drink dependency, a reformed alcoholic, and living proof that today's decision is tomorrow's freedom. Follow the expert advice contained here, and it will help you give up drinking – for good.

Living with Alzheimer's Disease and Similar Conditions
Dr Gordon Wilcock

This complete and compassionate self-help guide is designed for families and carers (professional or otherwise) faced with the 'living bereavement' of dementia.

Living with Stress
Cary L. Cooper, Rachel D. Cooper and Lynn H. Eaker

Stress leads to more stress, and the authors of this helpful book show why low levels of stress are desirable and how best we can achieve them in today's world. Looking at those most vulnerable, they demonstrate ways of breaking the vicious circle that can ruin lives.

READ MORE IN PENGUIN

A SELECTION OF HEALTH BOOKS

Living with Asthma and Hay Fever   John Donaldson

For the first time, there are now medicines that can prevent asthma attacks from taking place. Based on up-to-date research, this book shows how the majority of sufferers can beat asthma and hay fever to lead full and active lives.

Anorexia Nervosa   R. L. Palmer

Lucid and sympathetic guidance for those who suffer from this disturbing illness and their families and professional helpers, given with a clarity and compassion that will make anorexia more understandable and consequently less frightening for everyone involved.

Medicines: A Guide for Everybody   Peter Parish

The use of any medicine is always a balance of benefits and risks – this book will help the reader understand how to extend the benefits and reduce the risks. Completely revised, it is written in ordinary, accessible language for the layperson, and is also indispensable to anyone involved in health care.

Other People's Children   Sheila Kitzinger

Though step-families are common, adults and children in this situation often feel isolated because they fail to conform to society's idealized picture of a normal family. This sensitive, incisive book is essential reading for anyone involved with or in a step-family.

Miscarriage   Ann Oakley, Ann McPherson and Helen Roberts

One million women worldwide become pregnant every day. At least half of these pregnancies end in miscarriage or stillbirth. But each miscarriage is the loss of a potential baby, and that loss can be painful to adjust to. Here is sympathetic support and up-to-date information on one of the commonest areas of women's reproductive experience.

READ MORE IN PENGUIN

A SELECTION OF HEALTH BOOKS

When a Woman's Body Says No to Sex   Linda Valins

Vaginismus – an involuntary spasm of the vaginal muscles that prevents penetration – has been discussed so little that many women who suffer from it don't recognize their condition by its name. Linda Valins's practical and compassionate guide will liberate these women from their fears and sense of isolation and help them find the right form of therapy.

Mixed Messages   Brigid McConville

Images of breasts – young and naked, sexual and chic – are everywhere. Yet for many women, the form, functions and health of our own breasts remain shrouded in mystery, ignorance – even fear. The consequences of our culture's breast taboos are tragic: Britain's breast-cancer death rate is the highest in the world. Every woman should read *Mixed Messages* – the first book to consider the well-being of our breasts in the wider contexts of our lives.

Defeating Depression   Tony Lake

Counselling, medication, and the support of friends can all provide invaluable help in relieving depression. But if we are to combat it once and for all, we must face up to perhaps painful truths about our past and take the first steps forward that can eventually transform our lives. This lucid and sensitive book shows us how.

Freedom and Choice in Childbirth   Sheila Kitzinger

Undogmatic, honest and compassionate, Sheila Kitzinger's book raises searching questions about the kind of care offered to the pregnant woman – and will help her make decisions and communicate effectively about the kind of birth experience she desires.

The Complete New Herbal   Richard Mabey

The new bible for herb users – authoritative, up-to-date, absorbing to read and hugely informative, with practical, clear sections on cultivation and the uses of herbs in daily life, nutrition and healing.

READ MORE IN PENGUIN

A SELECTION OF HEALTH BOOKS

Twins, Triplets and More Elizabeth Bryan

This enlightening study of the multiple birth phenomenon covers all aspects of the subject from conception and birth to old age and death. It also offers much comfort and support as well as carefully researched information gained from meeting several thousands of children and their families.

Meditation for Everybody Louis Proto

Meditation means liberation from stress, anxiety and depression. This lucid and readable book by the author of *Self-Healing* describes a variety of meditative practices. From simple breathing exercises to more advanced techniques, there is something here to suit everybody's needs.

Endometriosis Suzie Hayman

Endometriosis is currently surrounded by many damaging myths. Suzie Hayman's pioneering book will set the record straight and provide both sufferers and their doctors with the information necessary for an improved understanding of this frequently puzzling condition.

The New Our Bodies, Ourselves
The Boston Women's Health Book Collective

To be used by all generations, *The New Our Bodies, Ourselves* courageously discusses many difficult issues, and is tailored to the needs of women in the 1990s. It provides the most complete advice and information available on women's health care. This British edition is by Angela Phillips and Jill Rakusen.

Not On Your Own Sally Burningham
The MIND Guide to Mental Health

Cutting through the jargon and confusion surrounding the subject of mental health to provide clear explanations and useful information, *Not On Your Own* will enable those with problems – as well as their friends and relatives – to make the best use of available help or find their own ways to cope.